MEN AT RISK

Men at Risk

Masculinity, Heterosexuality, and HIV Prevention

Shari L. Dworkin

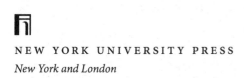

NEW YORK UNIVERSITY PRESS

New York and London

NEW YORK UNIVERSITY PRESS
New York and London
www.nyupress.org

References to Internet websites (URLs) were accurate at the time of writing. Neither the author nor New York University Press is responsible for URLs that may have expired or changed since the manuscript was prepared.

ISBN: 978-1-4798-0645-4 (hardback)
ISBN: 978-0-8147-2076-9 (paperback)

For Library of Congress Cataloging-in-Publication data, please contact the Library of Congress.

New York University Press books are printed on acid-free paper, and their binding materials are chosen for strength and durability. We strive to use environmentally responsible suppliers and materials to the greatest extent possible in publishing our books.

Manufactured in the United States of America

10 9 8 7 6 5 4 3 2 1

Also available as an ebook

CONTENTS

ACKNOWLEDGMENTS

This book would not have been possible without the help and hard work of so many people. I am very grateful to Dean Peacock and his team at Sonke Gender Justice and to Chris Colvin at the University of Cape Town for their collegiality, comments, collaboration, and incredible contributions to the field of masculinity studies, gender relations, violence, and HIV prevention, treatment, and care. I am also grateful to Abbey Hatcher, MPH, who was a research scientist and program coordinator for the South Africa data collection process. She carried out an extraordinary amount of work and was very involved in the coding and analysis of the data set. She also participated in the training of our interviewers in Cape Town, South Africa, for several days. Our interviewers for the South Africa portion of this project—Thomas Mogale, Richard Manamela, and Nkuli Ndlovu—were simply extraordinary in their skills and abilities, and they deeply probed very challenging issues with great respect, care, and sensitivity. They also transcribed all of our interview data into the local language and then into English. I thank them for that, and in particular I thank Nkuli, who examined and contributed to drafts of a paper from this study.

I am grateful to the University of California–San Francisco (UCSF) School of Nursing for offering a pilot award that supported the data collection in this book. I am also appreciative of the Center for AIDS Research (CFAR) UCSF Gladstone Institute of Virology and Immunology for providing funds for the pilot study "Laying the Groundwork to Test a Science-Based HIV and Violence Prevention Intervention among Heterosexually Active Men in South Africa," which is where the data from the second sample came from for chapter 4 of this book. I also am very grateful to the Whitely Center in Friday Harbor, Washington, where I worked over the course of several writing retreats to complete this manuscript. Their acceptance of my application to work at that location meant uninterrupted time in which to work, and the surroundings there were truly lovely, silent, and conducive to writing.

I acknowledge that all of my advisors and mentors over the years since 1992 have each contributed something quite central to my thinking, and I thank all of them from the University of Maryland, the University of Southern California, and Columbia University. I am indebted to the Department of Sociology at the University of California–San Diego and the Department of Social and Behavioral Sciences at UCSF for allowing me to present my work in a forum that was incredibly constructive and helpful to my thinking. And I reserve, of course, the most thanks to my partner, Kari Lerum, who is so brilliant, funny, and loving—and was so incredibly patient with me while I sat for absurd amounts of time and didn't offer my usual emotional presence to her. She inspires me intellectually and creatively each and every day of my life, and without her, this book would not be possible.

Finally, this book is also the result of an enormous amount of research, writing, and thinking that I have been doing since the year 2004. Portions of the chapters in this book are based on the following published articles, and I have expanded upon all of this previous work: Dworkin 2005; Dworkin & Blankenship 2009; Dworkin, Fullilove, & Peacock 2009; Dworkin 2010; Dworkin, Dunbar, Krishnan, Hatcher, & Sawires 2011; Dworkin, Colvin, Hatcher, & Peacock 2012; Dworkin, Hatcher, Colvin, & Peacock 2013; Higgins, Hoffman, & Dworkin, 2010. For the Dworkin et al. 2011 publication, the copyright holder is the American Public Health Association, and the full citation is Dworkin, S. L., Dunbar, M. S., Krishnan, S., Hatcher, A. M., & Sawires, S. (2011). Uncovering tensions and capitalizing on synergies in HIV/AIDS and antiviolence programs. *American Journal of Public Health, 101*, 995–1003.

1

Masculinity and HIV/AIDS Prevention

Heterosexually Active Men as the "Forgotten Group"?

Although the first AIDS cases in the United States were attributed to men having sex with men, over 70% of HIV infections worldwide and nearly one out of three new infections in the United States are now estimated to occur through sex between women and men (CDC 2013a; UNAIDS 2012). Globally, while there is wide regional variation in the percentage of cases attributable to sex between women and men, one thing is clear: the proportion of women with HIV is rising in many regions of the world. In Asia, women are 30% of those living with HIV, and in sub-Saharan Africa, the percentage of adults living with HIV who are women is 60%. It is vital to note that increases in the proportion of women with HIV have occurred in a relatively short period of time; globally, in 1985, 30% of infected people were women, and this percentage now stands at approximately 50%.

Even in the United States, where the main group affected by HIV and AIDS is men who have sex with men (MSM), sex between women and men is now by far the main means of transmission for women and is the second most prevalent means of transmission for men. This is different from what HIV/AIDS transmission looked like in the past in the United States. In earlier stages of the epidemic in the United States, intravenous drug use (IDU) was the second most common means of transmission for men, and IDU was the main means of transmission for women. Among women diagnosed in the United States, sex with a man as the identified source of transmission more than tripled from 1985 to the present, and the Centers for Disease Control now regularly reports that 86% of cases of HIV among women are categorized as being from exposure to "high-risk heterosexual contact" (CDC 2013a). "Heterosexual sex" now accounts for 28% of all new infections in the United States; that is, one in five new HIV infections is among women who are infected through sex with a man, and approximately one in ten new infections is among men who are infected through heterosexual sex (CDC 2013a, 2012). Combined, these facts underscore that sexual behavior change not just among women but also among heterosexually active men will be key to controlling the HIV epidemic for both men and women. Unfortunately, this emphasis in HIV prevention has been sorely lacking, both domestically and globally.

Let's examine the situation from another angle—first, globally. Approximately 30.7 million adults are living with HIV, and women constitute approximately 50% of the people living with HIV/AIDS globally. That is, of the 35.3 million people living with HIV (adults plus children), women constitute 17.7 million cases, children under fifteen years account for 3.3 million HIV cases, and adults are 32.1 million of the 35.3 million (UNAIDS 2012). Thus, if within the global pandemic, half of those who are infected are women, who is the other half? The other half is men, and globally, the large majority of cases are acquired through sex between women and men. However, the words "heterosexually active men" are not mentioned much in numerous national and key multilateral or bilateral agency reports. This is the case even in UNAIDS reports, and UNAIDS is the joint United Nations response to HIV and AIDS globally.

Discourses about "risk" and "vulnerability" that will be critically examined in this book circulate throughout numerous public arenas as a result of UNAIDS reports, and, interestingly, in the key surveillance slides, "women," "children," and "adults" are listed, but men are not. In fact, within the global surveillance slides at UNAIDS, men who have sex with men are often mentioned, but heterosexually active men and bisexually active men are not. Understandably, some men who have sex with men—or who have sex with both men and women—do not reveal this to others, and hence they may be difficult to identify or count. Additionally, homophobia and biphobia lead to a lack of recognition of men who have sex with men and men who have sex with women and men, leading to a lack of surveillance mechanisms being put in place in several countries to count such men (although 64 countries reported MSM as a surveillance category in 2010 and 104 countries reported MSM in 2012 [UNAIDS 2012]). Even though plenty of men worldwide have sex with both women and men (Dodge et al. 2012; Weinberg, Williams, & Pryor

1994), no country has a surveillance category for men who have sex with both women and men. Surveillance problems aside, however, currently, the large majority of HIV cases are said to be transmitted between a woman and a man. And yet, heterosexually active men in science-based prevention ("science-based" prevention efforts in this book refer to interventions funded by the National Institutes of Health and the Centers for Disease Control) efforts are often forgotten—both domestically and globally (except for international male circumcision efforts).

It is quite striking that heterosexually active men in the United States, particularly Black heterosexually active men—who are by far the most affected by HIV—have even been referred to by the National Association for the Advancement of Colored People (NAACP) and the National Action network (which works to serve Black communities in the United States) as "forgotten" by national and community-based HIV-prevention efforts (Raj et al. 2013). Nationally, it is true that the largest exposure category for the transmission of HIV is sex between men, but it is critical to look at regional variation concerning that trend. New surveillance data from the northeastern United States underscores that heterosexual transmission is the dominant mode of HIV acquisition for Black men (Raj & Bowleg 2012). Black men account for more than two-thirds of HIV cases that are classified as "heterosexual exposure" in the United States (Bowleg & Raj 2012). Shockingly, scrolling through the Centers for Disease Control (CDC) website in the United States reveals clear omissions concerning HIV risks among heterosexually active men. "Heterosexually active men" are not referenced under the "Who Is at Risk of HIV" section of the CDC website. Simultaneously, however, in 2010 on the CDC website, two authors ask in a short article whether there is a "generalized HIV epidemic" in various cities in America among Black MSM and Black heterosexuals (Dening & DiNenno 2010). Let me be clear: making mention of a possible "generalized epidemic" is a sign of a very serious epidemic—this is a term previously used to describe numerous developing countries experiencing an exacerbated HIV epidemic that has spread beyond sex workers, drug users, and men who have sex with men. If there is a near-generalized epidemic in parts of urban America "among Black MSM and Black heterosexuals," how could heterosexually active men not even be explicitly mentioned as an "at-risk" group?

Similarly, the new National HIV/AIDS Policy (Office of National AIDS Strategy 2010) is next to completely silent on the need to focus on heterosexually active men. The rationale is that because of limited resources, scarce dollars are being put into working with those groups that have "the highest" need, and thus the focus is on MSM. All of the above tells us that prevention with heterosexually active men risks being forgotten. This is startling not only for men but also because sex between a woman and a man accounts for 90% of new infections for Black women, 86% of new infections for Latina women, and 74% of new infections for White women (CDC 2013e).

The global UNAIDS reports aren't much better. Heterosexually active men are only mentioned in a few places in a several-hundred-page UNAIDS report where HIV/AIDS prevention is discussed. This is despite the fact that "unprotected heterosexual intercourse" is globally recognized as the "main mode" of HIV transmission in many countries around the world, including sub-Saharan Africa, the Caribbean, the Sudan, Papa New Guinea, most countries of Central Europe, and more. Despite this, it is the 2008 Global UNAIDS report that had the most material—only four paragraphs—that were dedicated specifically to prevention with heterosexually active men. Heterosexually active men are conflated with heterosexuality in that report (we do not know their sexual identities or the link between identities and practices because the surveillance mechanisms classify risks by behaviors, not identities). And, the 2012 version of the UNAIDS report no longer even includes a section from earlier reports on "tailored prevention for heterosexual men," wherein UNAIDS authors overtly examine the lack of adequate prevention with heterosexually active men by underscoring that

> while various prevention models have been developed to provide focused prevention support for men who have sex with men, few HIV prevention programmes have been specifically designed to take into account the values heterosexual men attach to sex, the pleasures they derive from it, and the social pressures associated with sex. A cardinal rule of HIV prevention is that programmes must be culturally relevant to the target population, but this maxim has not been rigorously followed among programmes that ostensibly aim to affect men's behaviours. (UNAIDS 2008, 121)

As domestic and global HIV epidemics progress, discourses of "vulnerability" and "risk" tend to be used within the same unquestioned frameworks that link gender and sexuality in very particular ways, as will be explained throughout this book. If countries do recognize gender relations as central to the spread of the epidemic, science-based prevention programs largely conflate gender with women and focus on women. When programs are designed for women, these are conceptualized in terms of women needing interventions to protect them from gender inequality, from passive female sexual negotiations, and from the behaviors of male partners. But in this conceptualization of the gender order, heterosexually active men—who are very often also race and class marginalized—need . . . what? What kinds of programming do heterosexually active men need to prevent HIV? Are heterosexually active men considered in prevention programs in the science base (outside of biomedical male circumcision programs or pre- and post-exposure prophylaxis)? When HIV prevention programs are carried out with heterosexually active men in the science base, do these programs make much-needed connections among race, class, masculinities, and sexuality in order to intervene in men's HIV risks? Are there structural domestic and global interventions for heterosexually active men designed to intervene in men's HIV risks when we know that structural drivers shape not only women's but also men's HIV risks (see chapter 2 for in-depth coverage of this point)?

Contrast this with the way heterosexually active women are framed within prevention programs and the way intervention programs are designed for women in the HIV pandemic. Analyses as to why women are at risk of HIV and AIDS both domestically and globally have been resoundingly clear: gender relations and gender inequality in particular have been identified as major "root causes" of what shapes and exacerbates the inception and course of the epidemic globally (Dworkin & Ehrhardt 2007; Gupta 1994, 2001, 2002; Gupta & Weiss 1993; Luke 2003; Kmietowicz 2004; UNAIDS 2008, 2012; Weiss & Gupta 1998). The above facts are said to be structural (e.g., lower levels of education and of access to the occupational structure, lower wages, lack of access to credit, lack of land ownership, property rights violations, food insecurity) but also have social and interpersonal dimensions (e.g., gendered power differentials, cultural devaluations of women, violence, trust, desire for closeness in relationships and in sex), and programs in HIV prevention therefore should work to "adequately address the contextual issues of heterosexual relationship dynamics" both domestically and globally (Logan, Cole, & Leukefield 2002, 873).

In the United States, the women most affected by HIV are Black women, whose rate of HIV infections is twenty times that of White women (CDC 2014). Black women's HIV risks are shaped by many of the gendered dynamics listed above, but they are also impacted by unique experiences of racial inequality, residential segregation, poverty, unemployment, men's incarceration histories, and a limited pool of available men (due to oppressive policing practices, poverty, incarceration). That is, in addition to the "gendered" factors mentioned above, the structural lack of availability of men can shape relationship dynamics, and research therefore finds that Black women are more likely to accept a lack of condom use and infidelity because of the desire to have and maintain a relationship with a male partner (Kline, Kline, & Okin 1992; McNair & Prather 2004; Newsome & Airhihenbuwa 2013).

Overall, then, while it seems abundantly clear at first glance that the centrality of "heterosexual relationship dynamics" means that both women and men need to be taken into account in science-based HIV/AIDS-prevention interventions, this has not historically been the case. That fact is the focus of this text. Why are women still the overwhelming focus of behavioral HIV-prevention interventions for "heterosexually active" adults in the science base, what has been the progression of (conceptual and empirical) work with heterosexually active men both domestically and globally, and what are the promises and limitations of past and current prevention programs with heterosexually active men? What should be done next? These are the main topics in this book.

Readers might still wonder, are heterosexually active men really even "vulnerable" to HIV? Does a discourse of vulnerability (with all of its attendant problems, which will be covered in chapter 2) that applies so easily to women and MSM even apply to heterosexually active men? And if so, does it apply to all heterosexually active men equally? How do we talk about heterosexually active men as vulnerable to HIV at the same time that we view men as race and class oppressed—and as participants in a gender order who may benefit from relationship power, male sexual entitlements, and other power differentials that shape women's

HIV risks (see chapters 2, 3, and 5)? What are the promises and limitations of HIV-prevention interventions that focus solely on gendered power and women's empowerment to reduce women's HIV/AIDS risks but do not focus on men at all (chapter 3)?

How should HIV/AIDS-prevention research proceed with a simultaneous understanding that women are disproportionately affected by the HIV/AIDS epidemic due to gender, race, and class inequalities and therefore require empowerment but that heterosexually active men and their health are also harmed by these factors (chapters 2–5)? How shall we as researchers and practitioners ensure that gender norms are viewed as playing a role in HIV transmission for heterosexually active men? Can this view occur alongside the view that recognizes that men are also harmed by structural inequalities such as racism, unemployment, heterosexism, oppressive policing practices, the prison system, migratory systems, processes of globalization, war, conflict, and more—and that these inequalities shape men's HIV-risk behaviors (chapters 2, 3, and 4)? In rare cases where HIV-prevention programming actively attempts to wrestle with the many complex social forces that shape men's HIV risks (globally), what is the result in terms of impacting gender relations, HIV risks, and violence (chapter 4)? Where programs do focus on gender relations as a root cause of HIV transmission, do men in prevention programs embrace global health programming trends that ask them to challenge gendered power relations in the name of improved health? Or do heterosexually active men resist such calls, viewing themselves as disempowered by race and class and equating calls for gender equality in health programs with a loss of masculine authority (chapter 4)?

These are the main questions posed in this text, but there are others that are relevant. How, for example, shall prevention researchers simultaneously wrestle with the recognition that women's social and structural empowerment is an important project in HIV/AIDS prevention—while also recognizing that masculinity, sex, and sexuality, defined according to constructs of "heterosexual identity," tend to structure sex according to a hydraulic model of male desire, the predominance of penile-vaginal penetration, the centrality of male pleasure, and masculinity as bolstered by multiple partners (Flood 2003a, 2003b; Holland et al. 1994a, 1994b; Kimmel 1995; Vittelone 2000)? How exactly is HIV prevention to succeed when male condoms are overwhelmingly reported by men as decreasing pleasure and sensations (Choi, Rickman, & Catania 1994; Conley & Collins 2005; Khan et al. 2004) and when some feminist researchers have now pointed out that women increasingly report the same (Pulerwitz & Dworkin 2006; Higgins 2007; Higgins & Hirsch 2008)? On top of this, outside of biomedical solutions to HIV prevention (e.g., male circumcision, microbicide candidate products for anal and vaginal use, pre-exposure prophylaxis, or "PREP"), female condoms are "the only alternative to the male condom as a means of protection against both pregnancy and STDs," and female condoms are not even adequately distributed or promoted in many countries while negative provider attitudes prevail and do not receive adequate intervention (Hoffman et al. 2004).

Throughout this book, it will be necessary for me to engage with the tensions between lines of work that focus on challenging oppressive gender relations in the name of HIV risk reduction and those lines of work that focus on masculinities and heterosexually active men to prevent HIV. I will pay special attention to the profoundly popular "vulnerability" paradigm in HIV research that portrays only women—and not heterosexually active men—as being "vulnerable" to HIV. I will critique this model and argue that it (vulnerable woman/invulnerable man) privileges gender analysis while omitting the unmarked category (men) and looks mainly at hegemonic definitions of masculinity while negating race and class marginalization. Ultimately, I will delve into how the current focus on "gendered" HIV-prevention interventions erases important drivers of HIV transmission—and therefore erases, marginalizes, or renders less fathomable or even unfathomable some important solutions to the HIV epidemic. Drawing on a "vulnerability" model, HIV prevention programs often seek to encourage women to employ more assertive sexual negotiations, but this model tends to ascribe men's HIV infection to their participation in a system of gender oppression that privileges men and harms women. This negates the fact that some men are at much greater risk of HIV infection than others, that men are not only beneficiaries in a system of gender relations but also experience harm in it (Courtenay 2000a, 2000b, 2000c; Messner 1997), and that, if there are disjunctures between men's sexual identity and sexual acts, this may shape their own and women's HIV risks.

At the same time, this book will recognize that paying attention to the ways in which heterosexually active men are harmed through the gender order and in the HIV/AIDS epidemic is not some sort of antifeminist, relativistic, "equal-opportunity harm" argument, but rather that studying men and masculinity in the HIV/AIDS epidemic is, similar to studying men and masculinity in many other realms and disciplines, a feminist enterprise. It requires the ability to attend to hierarchies in an institutionally supported system of gender relations where men as a group benefit over and above women as a group and where women are disproportionately harmed (Connell 1987, 1995a; Messner 1997). But it also requires simultaneous examination of the "costs to masculinity"—recognition that both men and women are harmed when men adhere to narrow and restrictive definitions of manhood (Connell 1995a; Messner 1997).

It is important to recognize that studying men and masculinity in the HIV/AIDS epidemic also requires drawing on the critical insights of multiracial feminist studies, which have already pointed out that women are not a homogenous group and thus, men aren't either (Baca-Zinn & Thornton Dill 1993; Cole 2009; Crenshaw 1991; Hill-Collins 1986, 1990; hooks 1984, 2000). These insights can press HIV researchers to then think about how some men disproportionately pay the health and inequality harms of the gender order—and how this affects both women's and men's health. Such thinking also requires that researchers consider the social and structural aspects of constraints on men's behaviors, just as they do with women, and not essentialize individual "problematic" behaviors as being the cause of harm to men or to women. Thus, in addition to furthering the call to bolster the study of masculinity within the field of HIV/AIDS prevention, I will put forward multiracial feminist calls for intersectionality (the simultaneous intersection of gender, race, class, and sexuality: Baca-Zinn & Thornton Dill 1993; Crenshaw 1991; Hill-Collins 1986, 1990, 1999) that I consider to be urgent in the area of global and public health concerning matters related to men, women, HIV/AIDS transmission, and HIV/AIDS prevention (see chapters 2, 4, and 5).

Let me be clear: we are in the fourth decade of the epidemic in the United States, where the dynamics of gender, race, class, and sexuality relations intersect to produce sex between women and men as the largest category of transmission in the world, and yet heterosexually active men are not often intervened with in the HIV/AIDS-prevention science base because they are not seen as having gender or as being affected by masculinity and gender relations—or as being impacted by race and class inequalities. All of these factors are not often intervened upon in the HIV-prevention-intervention science base with heterosexually active men (for a few domestic exceptions, see a systematic review by Dworkin, Treves-Kagan, & Lippman 2013). For this particular author, this omission is very difficult to understand.

Some might argue that the focus on women must be retained and that a focus on men is not a feminist enterprise. But how could this not be a feminist enterprise? The HIV literature has been wholly inspired by feminist thought on gendered power relations and sexuality and has already found (a) that worldwide, women's greatest risk of HIV comes from their male partner, often their husband (Glynn et al. 2001, 2003; Hirsch et al. 2007); (b) that violence is highly associated with HIV and that globally, women experience unprecedented amounts of violence (Beadnell et al. 2000; Dunkle et al. 2004, 2006; El-Bassel et al. 2004; Gruskin et al. 2002; Heise 1995; Jewkes, Levin, & Penn-Kekana 2003; Jewkes, Dunkle, et al. 2006, Jewkes et al. 2010, 2011; Lang et al. 2013; O'Toole, Shiffman, & Kiter-Edwards 2007; Maman et al. 2002; Messner & Stevens 2002; Silverman et al. 2008; UNAIDS 2012; Watts & Zimmerman 2002; WHO 2000, 2004, 2005, 2013; Wingood & DiClemente 1996, 2000, 2002; Zierler 1997); (c) that men generally have the right to initiate and expect sex and women are not frequently supposed to know as much about or to initiate sex (Crawford, Kippax, & Waldby 1994; Dworkin & O'Sullivan 2005, 2010; Exner et al. 2003; Ortiz-Torres, Williams, & Ehrhardt 2003; Williams et al. 2001); (d) that men generally receive higher, not lower, status from having sex with multiple partners, women are often expected to be monogamous in a sexual double standard (Exner et al. 2003; Rutter & Schwartz 2011), and where women are not monogamous, they do not receive higher status from having sex with multiple partners (Egan 2013; Rutter & Schwartz 2011); and (e) that the structure of sexuality and gender relations in many regional contexts means that women will often not have as much of a voice in sexual matters or in several other household, familial, family planning, or relationship decisions, with much variation depending on the region (Dudgeon & Inhorn 2004; Gupta 1994, 2005). If these claims are as true as the feminist literature tells us, then it is very hard to understand why an analysis of men and masculinity has not been made central to preventing the

HIV epidemic among heterosexually active women and men. It is also very hard to understand why working with men from an intersectional perspective that takes structural race, class, and gender inequalities into account hasn't been a central part of the HIV-prevention solution from its inception to the present (Dworkin 2005).

These topics are the focus of this text, which has the main goal of using sociology to carry out a critical public health analysis across the chapters in order to (a) underscore how, why, and with what consequences heterosexually active men have been so infrequently considered in science-based behavioral HIV-prevention efforts within the worst pandemic of our time; (b) challenge the notion that heterosexually active men are not "vulnerable" to HIV and provide much evidence for how they are epidemiologically, socially, and culturally "at risk," particularly when an intersectional analysis is used; (c) critically assess how there have been two tracks of work that operate separately—gendered power and "women's empowerment" programming and "work with men" to reduce HIV and violence risks (Here, I not only point out that separate tracks of work are operating but also examine the positive and negative overt and inadvertent consequences of keeping work centered on "women only" or "men only."); (d) drawing on empirical data that I collected in South Africa in collaboration with the University of Cape Town and Sonke Gender Justice (a South African NGO dedicated to working with heterosexually active men to reduce the spread and impact of HIV and work to reduce violence against both women and men), examine some promising new health programs in the arena of masculinities, gender equality, HIV/AIDS prevention, and antiviolence (Here, I will underscore some of the main successes and challenges of carrying out such work.); and (e) propose, from disciplines outside of public-health HIV studies (such as sociology, masculinity studies, gender-relations studies, and medical sociology), some guidance for and direction to the field of behavioral HIV prevention.

To be sure, there have been many journal articles on heterosexually active men and HIV "risk" (but not much on heterosexually active men and HIV prevention) and a few chapters of books on the topic of sexuality, masculinity, and HIV. For example, Catherine Waldby, in *AIDS and the Body Politic: Biomedicine and Sexual Difference* (1996), examines why AIDS discourse in epidemiology and immunology produces gay men and women as "high-risk" categories, and other books have also carried out critical epidemiology, such as Cindy Patton's *Inventing AIDS* (1990) and *Globalizing AIDS* (2002) and Paula Treichler's *How to Have Theory in an Epidemic* (1999). In the edited volume titled *AIDS: Setting a Feminist Agenda* (Doyal, Naidoo, & Wilton 1994), where the focus is on explicating the links between feminist theory and HIV/AIDS risks among women, nearly the whole book is on women and HIV except for a chapter by Holland et al. (1994b), who examine the links between masculinity and sexuality in heterosexuality. Gary Barker's 2005 *Dying to Be Men* has a chapter on sexuality and sexual risk among men who have sex with women, and some of Carole Campbell's book *Women, Families, and the HIV Epidemic: A Sociological Perspective on the Epidemic in America* (1999) contains an examination of the domestic epidemic wherein she underscores that the focus of prevention should not rest on the shoulders of women alone. Jennifer Hirsch and her colleagues' edited anthropological volume *The Secret: Love, Marriage, and HIV* (2010) focuses on moving away from examining individual behavior within studies of sexuality and HIV and towards addressing the sexual-opportunity structures that produce male infidelity.

However, shockingly, no full-length sociological, social-scientific, or critical global-health manuscript (the latter is a newer field; see, e.g., Biehl & Petryna 2013) has examined masculinity and HIV-prevention programming among heterosexually active men. No full-length book has focused on what science-based researchers in the HIV prevention field have—and have not—designed and implemented with heterosexually active men. No full-length manuscript has critically examined what the promises and limitations of this body of work are, both domestically and globally. No book-length manuscript to date has examined how, despite the fact that gender relations and gender inequality are recognized to be main drivers of the HIV pandemic, analyses of men and masculinity rarely structure evidence-based prevention programs around the globe. Nor have books critically assessed how prevention programming with men has generally not been implemented as "gender-specific" (recognizing the different needs of women and men in programming or recognizing the specific ways in which gender relations shape HIV) or "gender-transformative" (attempting to intervene on structural inequalities and/or democratize gender relations in the name of improved health) (for an exception in the international realm, see chapter 4). No book has pondered and explained why, domestically, in 2013, the United States has only *one* NIH-funded, structurally informed HIV-prevention intervention for heterosexually active men that takes race and class inequalities into account (the program is covered in Raj et al. 2013).

At this point, let's step back a bit to consider how the field of HIV prevention arrived at this place and think about why these trends are occurring, not only in the interdisciplinary field of HIV/AIDS studies but also in other health realms (e.g., family planning and reproductive health). The goal of the remainder of this chapter is to trace the development of work on heterosexually active men in these other fields, lay out a theoretical framework that undergirds many HIV-prevention programs (the sex-gender-sexuality triad), and define the terms associated with the sex-gender-sexuality triad that will be commonly referred to (and challenged) throughout the book.

For the sake of definitions, it is important to offer a brief explanation of the terms "masculinity," "sex," "gender," "sexuality," and the "sex-gender-sexuality triad," as these will be some of the key terms used across the chapters. It is difficult to write about masculinity without writing about feminist perspectives on masculinities that view masculinities as constructed, as situated in regional and local histories and social relations, and as the products of institutional, interpersonal, individual, and cultural relations of power (Kaufman 1994; Kimmel 1987, 1990; Messner 1990, 2002). One of the most well-worn and frequently deployed concepts of masculinity within global health and public health has come from the social sciences and is hegemonic masculinity, which refers to the most dominant form of masculinity in a given era in a given time (usually White, middle-class, cisgender, and heterosexual) (Connell 1987; Messner 1997). Hegemonic masculinity is not meant to represent what an individual man is; rather, it represents an ideal that collectively structures a field of gender relations. Hegemonic masculinity is hierarchically defined in relation to subordinated and marginalized masculinities (working-class, gay, bisexual or transgender, minority, and/or poor men) and to women (Connell 1995a; Connell & Messerschmidt 2005). While a very small number of men might adhere to the norms and practices of hegemonic masculinity, this idealized version of masculinity helps to shape beliefs and social practices among many different groups of men (Connell & Messerschmidt 2005, 836; Morrell, Jewkes, & Lindegger 2012).

In this book, I not only draw on the concepts of hegemonic and subordinated masculinities, but I also draw upon conceptions of gender as relational (Connell 1987; McKay 1997) (as not being defined solely by masculinities but being dependent on relational definitions of femininities), and of masculinities as socially constructed, as agentically deployed in situations of agency and constraint (by race, class, and more), and as shifting over time and locale (Hunter 2005; Kimmel 1987, 1990; Messner 1997). I also will draw on ideas about masculinity as historically constructed and locally configured, as something that is not about "fixed traits" but is achieved via interaction, is historically produced, is in flux, and is a collective practice (Connell & Messerschmidt 2005; Courtenay 2000a, 2000b; Lorber 1994; West & Zimmerman 1987). And, throughout the book, when I write about the links among masculinity, sexuality, and sexual practices, consideration will be given to anti-essentialist ideas, which recognize that the range of masculinities available to men is shaped by many broader social forces (essentialism is a stance that steps away from the idea that men have fixed traits such as a "naturally uncontrollable" sex drive that is driven by biology) (Flood 2003a, 2003b; Vittelone 2000).

Moving on to the pieces of the sex-gender-sexuality triad, then, "sex" under modern medicine has come to mean two distinct and oppositional beings known as biological males and females; it is no doubt a highly contested term (Butler 1993; Cooky & Dworkin 2013; Fausto-Sterling 2000; Karkazis et al. 2012; Jordan-Young 2010; Van Den Wingaard 1997), one that has a genealogy all its own (Foucault 1978, 1980). Laqueur has argued that the "two sex" model in which men are viewed as biologically and dichotomously different from and oppositional to women is a relatively recent phenomenon in history. For example, according to historians, a one-sex model used to exist prior to the Enlightenment, which occurred during the seventeenth and eighteenth centuries in Europe. Such a model emphasized matters of degree in the sex system and also emphasized similarities in the ways in which male and female infants emerged from the same embryonic tissues (Laqueur 1990). Here, women were viewed as having nearly the same reproductive organs as men, albeit inside the body in the form of the vagina and fallopian tubes instead of outside the body. Galen's understanding of sex, for example, took us in temporal terms from the toppling of Rome to the Renaissance, the Reformation, and well beyond where he examined textbooks that underscored that if one were to "turn outward the woman's, turn inward, so to speak, and you will find the same in both in every respect" (qtd. in Laqueur 1990, 5). And before the eighteenth century, bodies were not always described in terms of natural differences or dichotomies, but rather were described in terms of inherent fluidity and ambiguity (Laqueur 1990). In fact, the current two-sex system that characterizes and fascinates Western consciousness (and beyond) only emerged at the turn of the nineteenth century, when racialized, classed, sexualized, and gendered discourses and practices were deployed to restructure notions of difference, superiority, and inferiority (Laqueur 1990).

While there is in fact some scientific understanding that there is a spectrum of human types from the perspective of examining hormones, gonads, and a combination of external and internal genitalia (Fausto-Sterling 1985, 2000; Jordan-Young 2010), sex is very typically viewed in terms of dichotomously different biological, hormonal, and physiological aspects of being male or female. It is this more restrictive definition of sex that is the one most often deployed in HIV/AIDS-prevention interventions (e.g., women in HIV prevention are viewed under the rubric of experiencing biological vulnerabilities associated with their sex—and socially and structurally produced gender roles and gender inequality within heterosexual sexual relations).

"Gender," albeit another contested term, has come to mean, at least within much of second wave feminist theory, the social construction of what it means to be a man or woman. This particular conceptual maneuver served as an entirely understandable enterprise within second wave feminism amidst claims that "biology is destiny" (à la Freud)—that women are somehow biologically inferior and better suited to domestic and maternal life than to the public sphere, positions of leadership, or the institution of sport. As a result, uncoupling what was viewed as socially constructed gender from what was perceived as biological sex opened up the way for emancipation for some within the gender order (Friedan 1964; Lorber 1994). Gender concerns the ways in which roles, norms, behaviors, and self-presentations cohere as culturally produced expectations for a particular sex. In this way, gender can be viewed not as the fixed property of an individual nor as a fixed system of roles that rest on an essentialist sex base but rather as repeatedly produced in patterned interactions with others according to expectations, reward systems, societal valuations, and valued identities (West & Fenstermaker 1995; West & Zimmerman 1987). Much has been written on the way women's and men's roles and norms have shaped both sexuality and HIV risks in heterosexually active sex acts (see below, this chapter).

"Sexuality" in this text will refer to a continuum of sexual object choices (homosexual, bisexual, heterosexual, queer, and other options) that individuals and groups express in terms of both behavior and/or identities (DeLamater & Hyde 2007; Klein 1999; Stombler et al. 2009; Valocchi 2007). It also refers to a system of social relations that hierarchilizes relations between groups of people according to societal norms and values (i.e., heterosexuality tends to be more highly valued) (Rubin 1999). These definitions are referred to as constructionist, given their recognition that sexuality is not a "natural drive" or an essentialist force that is "expressed" in society but rather that social relations structure what we know as possibilities and how we understand sexual acts and identities as linked (or unlinked) within a particular sexual system (i.e., not a cause of nature, but an effect of power). Early constructionists included those such as Kinsey, who, in his groundbreaking works *Sexual Behavior in the American Male* (1948) and *Sexual Behavior in the American Female* (1953), underscored the range of sexual behaviors that U.S. citizens enacted. He found that 37% of American males in his sample had had a same-sex experience to orgasm, despite the fact that a very small percentage identified as gay. Similarly, he found that 13% of women in his study had had a same-sex experience to orgasm, despite the fact that a very small percentage identified as lesbian. The resultant "Kinsey" scale refers to the need to break away from three discrete identity categories (homosexual, bisexual, heterosexual) to consider a continuum of sexuality whereon very few people identify as predominantly heterosexual or predominantly homosexual, and there is recognition that identities and sexual acts may not match.

Foucault's (1978) work partly focused on the role that medicine and psychiatry play in constituting the realm of the fathomable, both discursively and in practice, concerning a binary of heterosexuality and homosexuality. This was groundbreaking for the study of sexuality. He argued that these categories, rather than reflecting natural realities, are discursive effects—products of power and knowledge. Instead of viewing sexuality in terms of deviant versus normal acts that have always existed throughout history, Foucault argued that the formation of sexual identities emerged with a broader shift in power relations whereby regimes of normalization regulated populations according to sexual personhood. Others agree that sexual-identity categories such as heterosexuality and homosexuality are relatively recent phenomena that emerged in the nineteenth century (Foucault 1978; Katz 1995; Weeks 1985, 2002), and this, alongside a reliance on conceptions of oppositional binaries, is in fact part of the reason why bisexuality and other categories were/are so late to make their way into and challenge a largely upheld dichotomy within the field of HIV prevention and beyond (Dodge, Reese, & Gebhard 2008; Muñoz-Laboy & Dodge 2005; Rodriguez-Rust 1999; Sandfort & Dodge 2008).

Several of the thinkers mentioned above (and many others) underscore two key features of the social organization of sexuality that are important considerations for this book. The first is that there can be a divergence between sexual identities and sexual acts and there need not be a one-to-one correspondence between the two. This is due to various social inequalities, individual preferences, or, more broadly, differences in sexual systems that prescribe the links between sexual acts and sexual identities across different regions (Almaguer 1990; Carillo 2002; Diaz 1998; Lang 1999; Lorber 1996; Parker 1999a, 1999b; Sandfort & Dodge 2008; Thing 2010). The second common element among the thinkers referred to above is the idea that sexuality is neither essential nor natural but is instead an emergent process that is shaped by social histories and is embedded within social interactions and relationships according to the structure of institutions and to the sex-gender-sexuality system of a given society. Far from being "natural" or "essential," sexuality is also immanently tied to race and class relations both domestically (Hill-Collins 2005; Mahay, Laumann, & Michaels 2001; Staples 2006; Thing 2010) and globally (Gevisser & Cameron 1995; Hoad, Martin, & Reid 2005; Hunter 2004, 2007; Swarr 2012). Thus, to be clear, this book is also part of an antiracist perspective that challenges notions of race- and class-marginalized men being essentially different from more racially dominant men. I argue that it is critical to understand historical and contemporary social relations, including structural and interpersonal race, class, and gender relations, in order to understand men's sexual practices.

While several of these ideas may be common sense to many social scientists, it is not common sense more broadly to view sex as anything but "natural," and it is not common sense to see that the linkages across the sex-gender-sexuality triad hinge upon factors other than biology. But such essentialist notions are not satisfying for scholars who are interested in the social construction of sexuality and the sexual construction of society (Connell & Dowsett 1999; Dowsett 1996; Epstein 1996; Lorber 1996, 1999; Katz 1995; Parker 1999a, 1999b; Rich 1982; Richardson 1996; Rubin 1999; Seidman 2009; Vance 1983, 1993; Valocci 2007; Weeks 1985, 2002). After all, it is difficult to make sense of the fact that kissing is seen as sexualized, "natural" foreplay to Americans and Europeans while it is virtually unknown among the Balinese, the Siriono of South America, the Thonga of Africa, and the Lepcha of Eurasia (Tiefer 1990). And we must wonder why it is that young men in Papua, New Guinea, believe that young boys needed to be inseminated with the semen of older men in order to grow into manhood while same-sex sexual experiences are not part of normative adolescent male scripts in the United States (Herdt 1993). How is it that the Greeks organized same-sex sexual relations not around a sex-gender-sexuality triad but around age structures and public status (Langlands 2006; Williams 1999)? Thus, the linkages that are made (or not) across the sex-gender-sexuality triad are due to an understanding of sexuality as socially structured, as institutionally and legally supported (or unsupported), and as requiring an understanding of local meanings—such systems are the effects of power: normalization, surveillance, repetition, and the interrelationships between discourse and practice (Foucault 1978).

The simple insight that there need not be a correspondence between sexual identity and sexual acts would have served as especially useful early in the HIV/AIDS epidemic, given that "heterosexual transmission" as it is now counted in the domestic or global epidemic may in fact mean that a bisexual man is having sex with a bisexual woman, or it may mean that a queer woman is having sex with a heterosexual man, according to the allowable categorizations. It can mean that a man who identifies as heterosexual (and does not disclose same-sex practices) but has sex with women and men will be classified as having "heterosexual" sex risks. Oddly enough, a gay woman could have sex with a gay man and her risk would be classified as "heterosexual sex." (These topics will be examined in more depth in chapter 2.) Within HIV/AIDS surveillance categories within the United States, the only options for transmission "risk" are "intravenous drug use," "men who have sex with men," and "heterosexual sex," and within the global epidemic, "sex workers," "drug users," "men who have sex with men," and "pregnant women" are commonly deployed terms. Since all cases of HIV are measured in surveillance mechanisms by sexual acts (e.g., men who have sex with men or heterosexual acts of sexual transmission), there are also challenges to erasures of sexual identity within these classifications (Young & Meyer 2005).

Definitions concerning the sex-gender-sexuality triad and assumed linkages within it are crucially important to consider for HIV prevention given conceptions around the world that the triad itself is a natural, essential force that differs categorically for women and men and is naturally heterosexual or homosexual (and occasionally bisexuality is recognized). As has been argued by other scholars, the "primary obstacle to a sociological understanding of sexuality" (Epstein 1996, 147) is that "rarely do we turn from consideration of the organs themselves to the sources of meaning that are attached to them, the ways in which the physical activities of sex are learned, and the ways in which these activities are integrated into larger social scripts and social arrangements where meaning and sexual behavior come together to create sexual conduct" (Gagnon & Simon 1963, 5, as cited in Epstein 1996, 147). This insight is also crucial for HIV/AIDS prevention to wrestle with, as researchers should not take for granted the common understanding that women and men have around the world concerning the male sex drive as biologically natural and uncontrollable (Holland et al. 1994b; Segal 1994; Vittelone 2000). Hence, acknowledging and unhinging the ways in which norms of masculinity interact with men's (and women's) essentialist understandings of their own bodies could be helpful in altering sexual decision making in HIV prevention.

Despite my own recognition of masculinity as historically and regionally constituted and specified and despite the way that I will be underscoring that masculine formations intersect with the sex-gender-sexuality triad of a given locale, much critique in this book will be centered on the most commonly deployed (normative) definitions of sex-gender-sexuality and their primary linkages as these are conceived within HIV/AIDS-prevention interventions. I am also aware that some readers will see the words "heterosexual sex," "heterosexual transmission," and "heterosexually identified" as reifications of what are not stable categories (or even helpful categories) that all too often may leave out bisexual populations—and I am aware that my comments about "sex" and "sexuality" and "men" and "women" will also be viewed by some as uncritically referring to cisgender (biologically born) women and men or as taking at face value a "heterosexual" identity where this may need to be challenged. Some might even be upset that I am muddying the category "heterosexual" by devoting any attention to men who identify as heterosexual but whose sexual practices are not solely with women. I am aware of these critiques and think these are very important and worthy points. In this book, my focus is on examining and challenging the most commonly deployed concepts in HIV-prevention interventions with heterosexually active men (recognizing that interventions with heterosexually active men may very well target individuals who have sex with both women and men or other configurations not recognized by the categories themselves).

For the purposes of this book, defining the terms "sex," "gender," and "sexuality" is especially crucial, as are the connections among these, partly because of the unique influence that second wave feminist thought has had on gender-related HIV prevention programming for both women and men. Second wave feminist thought generally linked women to a system of gender oppression within heterosexuality that was defined as the sex-gender system. As I will examine in chapter 2, there are two primary assumptions within the sex/gender system that were translated into much of second wave feminism during its rise in the academy from the 1960s to the 1990s. Over the last several decades, the same two assumptions have woven their way deeply into the HIV-prevention literature through ideas about "gender roles" and "heterosexual transmission." In this framework, given the assumption that heterosexually active men might be "perpetrators" in the epidemic, they were not necessarily viewed as "vulnerable" to HIV—and it may therefore not be a surprise that a parallel examination of male roles or male norms did not emerge early on in the HIV epidemic or within the field of prevention. Indeed "male roles" and "male norms" were conspicuously absent from the early analyses of HIV. Two of the first scholars to provide in-depth coverage of "male gender norms," sexuality, and HIV/AIDS were Tamsin Wilton and Peter Aggeleton in a talk on safer sex in Scandinavia (1990). In their talk, they "deplore" the "invisibility of the heterosexual male norm" in HIV and AIDS discourse, and Wilton (1994) argued that it is important not to focus solely on women's behavior but to change men's behavior because it is "men's behavior which puts women at risk" (Wilton 1994, 6). I will be elaborating on how this interpretation of HIV transmission is narrow because it assumes that male perpetration of HIV infection and of harms to women are the main ways to conceive of masculinity, sexuality, and HIV risks.

Analyses of men and masculinity were somewhat more thoroughly explored later by Carole Campbell (1995) in an article titled "Male Gender Roles and Sexuality: Implications for Women's AIDS Risk and Prevention." She argued that

> [b]y focusing singly on women, it [prevention] has ignored the role of men in sexual decision making and has reinforced the belief that women are responsible for safer sex. Public health's well-intentioned effort to warn women about their risk has simultaneously taken pressure off of men to practice safe behavior. While the attention to women's risk is important, it has perpetuated traditional beliefs about gender roles and thus has served to free men from taking responsibility for their own health and that of their female partners. The focus of prevention efforts on women is myopic in that women who represent one-half of a partnership are getting information but men who represent the other half are not.

She goes on to argue that

> [i]n recent years, despite attention to the special risk of women for HIV infection, AIDS cases among women continue to rise. . . . [T]his trend will continue until heterosexual men become the focus of prevention efforts. Therefore, this article calls attention to the need for a change in emphasis in AIDS prevention strategies targeted to heterosexuals in the U.S. This change must involve men as responsible for their health behavior and it must target men directly. (Campbell 1995, 198)

Consistent with my critique of work that sees men as perpetrators in the HIV epidemic, she remarks,

> A negative image of men is present . . . in AIDS prevention information. Perhaps in the lack of attention to men, there is an underlying assumption that men really do not care about safer sex practices and that men will not be motivated to change their behavior. Men are not treated as being responsive to health concerns, but instead as being uninterested and dependent on women. . . . Rather than directly targeting men as responsible individuals, AIDS prevention has given instructions to women on how to negotiate safer sex with their partners. (Campbell 1995, 205)

Campbell is a sociologist. And, approximately four years later, within the field of public health, those who design and implement evidence-based HIV/AIDS-prevention interventions also thought this lack was quite profound/problematic and their voices began to ring out in journal articles.

More Than a Decade Ago

In 2009, in an article in the *American Journal of Public Health* titled "Are HIV/AIDS Prevention Interventions with Heterosexually Active Men in the United States Gender Specific?" I highlighted that it had been approximately fifteen years earlier when Theresa Exner and her colleagues at the HIV Center for Clinical and Behavioral Studies at the New York State Psychiatric Institute and Columbia University in New York City had written an article in *AIDS & Behavior* titled "HIV Risk Reduction Interventions with Heterosexual Men: The Forgotten Group" (Exner et al. 1999). These authors underscored that "HIV risk reduction interventions targeting heterosexual risk are warranted, particularly in higher risk communities" and that "while many HIV risk reduction interventions have been focused among women, heterosexual men have less frequently been the focus of such efforts" (348). Exner and her colleagues continued, "yet it is imperative that heterosexually active men be included in strategic efforts to reduce heterosexual transmission because sexual behavior is dyadic and men are the partners of women" (348).

To examine the state of the prevention field, Exner and her colleagues reviewed HIV-prevention interventions from 1980 to 1998 that focus on reducing "heterosexual risk behavior" among North American men. They placed an important focus on interventions that sought to change a behavioral outcome that reduces "heterosexual risk." Of the twenty interventions that they found to meet rigorous methodological standards, seven were for intravenous drug use. Of the remaining thirteen, only three targeted men exclusively while the rest focused on women and men. At that time, calls were made to bolster efforts to include heterosexual men (Exner et al. 1999). There was a clear need to make gendered components of interventions more explicit, and to push prevention studies beyond informational and condom-skills-building approaches, which were criticized as being gender-neutral approaches.

More Than a Decade Later . . .

But more than a decade later, where did the field shift? Another systematic review was carried out in conjunction with ongoing efforts at the Centers for Disease Control (CDC) with the Diffusion of Effective Behavioral Interventions program (DEBI). DEBI is the largest centralized effort to package, disseminate, and replicate effective HIV/AIDS behavioral interventions in the United States. Lyles et al. (2007) carried out a systematic review of the intervention literature from 2000 to 2004, detailing the eighteen interventions that meet the criteria for best evidence. Of the six best-evidence interventions that were designed for sexual risk-reduction for heterosexually active HIV-negative adults, four were for women, two were for both women and men (one of these is focused on those receiving outpatient psychiatric care; the other focuses on couples communication), and none intervened only with heterosexually active men. One of the two interventions for both women and men focused on issues of gender norms and gendered power (e.g., women as disempowered and needing to assertively negotiate safer sex), and all of the women-only interventions focus on some aspects of gendered norms and gendered power and emphasize the need to infuse women with more safer-sex negotiating power vis-à-vis a male partner.

In the 2009 article that I wrote with Robert Fullilove and Dean Peacock in the *American Journal of Public Health*, we revealed that of the six best-evidence interventions, two interventions were gender neutral and neither was for heterosexually active men (Carey et al. 2004; Shain et al. 1999), two were gender sensitive (focused on the needs of men, but not necessarily working to change male gender norms or recognize the intersection of race, class, and masculinity) (Baker et al. 2004; Hobfoll et al. 2002), and two were a mix of gender sensitive and transformative (El Bassel et al. 2003; Ehrhardt et al. 2000; Ehrhardt et al. 2002) (but both of these are focused on women).

Notably, in all of the above comprehensive reviews—and even in a third one that was centered on heterosexually active men (Elwy et al. 2002)—despite the number of interventions directed at heterosexual adults, the word "masculinity" was not mentioned once, there was no coverage of the ways in which men have gender, and no mention was made of how masculinity and gender relations shape men's HIV risks. A failure to mention gender roles, gender inequality, masculinity, or gender relations even occurred in the write-up of studies that identified certain male-dominated occupations and occupational groups such as truck driving. Instead, these were written up as opportunities to reach "high-risk" men.

From Women to Gender

As I have previously argued (Dworkin, Fullilove, & Peacock 2009) but will elaborate on here, the facts described above about the conflation of gender with women while men are left out may not be wholly surprising. This is the case because public health and HIV as a field have only recently started to make an otherwise common and important disciplinary shift in the study of gender relations. This shift is one that moves away from the common conflation of gender with women and women's oppression to the recognition of gender relations, or the ways in which both women and men are affected by gender inequality. Such an emphasis is much needed given the way in which women and men are differently positioned in and affected by gender norms and gender inequality (Connell 1987; Messner 1997). This type of shift is also urgent since masculinity as a set of beliefs, a set of social practices, and an institutionally supported set of structures definitively shapes both men's and women's health outcomes (Courtenay 2000b: Sabo & Gordon 1995).

But this point requires more consideration, and such an emphasis is not without politics. Indeed, across various disciplines in the United States, there has been a shift from "women" to "gender"—and the debates that have circulated around these shifts have invoked reactions that will be similar to those occurring with a shift to a focus on gender relations within the field of HIV prevention. Some feminist thinkers argued that a change from "women" to "gender" as an analytic maneuver would decenter women from an analysis of oppression and dilute recognition of the marginalized status for which they had just been recognized. Others argued that resources would rush to men even though women's issues were still sorely underfunded. Still others saw an emphasis on the "harms" of gender to men as depoliticizing and relativizing harms to women without acknowledging that many men benefit from systems of gender inequality. Some scholars argued that when the shift to "gender" from "women" took hold, women would lose leadership positions and that many new leadership positions would go to men in various gender-equality and gender-equality-and-health organizations. Still others argued that the term "gender" emerged in part because it was viewed as more "objective" and "neutral" and because it distanced itself from "feminism." Here, in her groundbreaking article in 1986, Joan Scott argued in the *American Historical Review* that

> [i]n its simplest recent usage, "gender" is a synonym for "women." Any number of books and articles whose subject is women's history have, in the past few years, substituted "gender" for "women" in their titles. In some cases, this usage, though vaguely referring to certain analytic concepts, is actually about the political acceptability of the field. In these instances, the use of "gender" is meant to denote the scholarly seriousness of a work, for "gender" has a more neutral and objective sound than does "women." "Gender" seems to fit within the scientific terminology of social science and thus dissociates itself from the (supposedly strident) politics of feminism. (Scott 1986, 1056)

She goes on to argue that gender can and should be an analytic category of its own:

> It seems to me significant that the use of the word "gender" has emerged at a moment of great epistemological turmoil that takes the form, in some cases, of a shift from scientific to literary paradigms among social scientists (from an emphasis on cause to one on meaning, blurring genres of

inquiry, in anthropologist Clifford Geertz's phrase); and, in other cases, the form of debates about theory between those who assert the transparency of facts and those who insist that all reality is construed or constructed, between those who defend and those who question the idea that "man" is the rational master of his own destiny. In the space opened by this debate and on the side of the critique of science developed by the humanities, and of empiricism and humanism by post-structuralists, feminists have not only begun to find a theoretical voice of their own but have found scholarly and political allies as well. It is within this space that we must articulate gender as an analytic category. (Scott 1986, 1066)

Indeed, there has always been a politics to "adding men" into the gender-relations mix in several fields (Connell 1987; Dworkin et al. 2011; McKay 1997), and this has certainly played out within fields other than HIV prevention. There are important lessons to be learned, then, from the realms of family planning, reproductive health, violence programming, and other health-related programs of research that have attempted to tackle the issue of working with heterosexually active men. Within the field of reproductive health and family planning, early work did not include men and portrayed men,

either explicitly or implicitly, as relatively unconcerned and unknowledgeable about reproductive health. They have been seen primarily as impregnators of women, or as the cause of women's poor reproductive health outcomes through STI exposure, sexual violence, and physical abuse. In addition, they have been regarded (often rightly so) as formidable barriers to women's decision-making about fertility, contraceptive use, and health-care utilization. Indeed, some of these generalizations about men have been empirically demonstrated across cultures. Relative to women, men tend to have more sexual partners over their lives, are more likely to have multiple partners simultaneously, are more likely to pursue commercial sex, are more likely to have extra-partner sexual relations, and are more likely to commit an act of violence against women, adolescents, and other men. (Dudgeon & Inhorn 2004, 1381)

However, these earlier characterizations of men broke down when the authors examined the bulk of the research, which also showed that in examining some of these stereotypes in demographic research, Greene and Biddlecom (2000) show consistent exceptions to many of these generalizations. They find that (1) men may be more, equally, or less informed about contraceptives than women, (2) many men participate in birth control through male- and coital-dependent methods, (3) men's pronatalism varies, with average fertility preferences often differing little from women's and with wide variation between men from different regions, (4) men's dominance in reproductive decision-making varies, and may vary over the reproductive life-course of the couple, (5) men may not prevent women from covertly using contraceptives, and (6) men as well as women may have financial motives for sex, because children may legitimate partners' claims to one another's resources. (Dudgeon & Inhorn 2004, 1382)

Some scholars underscored the lessons concerning work with men that HIV/AIDS-prevention researchers could have garnered earlier from other fields, such as those of family planning and reproductive health, but did not:

Research has found that although men are interested in family planning, they do not want to learn about it from their wives. However, most men report that they learn this information from either their wives or friends. Men do not generally learn about family planning from health care professionals because of the focus of family planning on women. It does appear that the lack of family planning information and services for men, rather than a lack of interest on men's part, has prevented men from taking an active role. (Campbell 1995, 206)

Campbell went on to say that programs designed to reach men have been effective, and that

[f]amily planning programs learned that in order to be effective, it was necessary to involve males. These programs also found that men were actually interested in getting information but did not have access to it. It does not appear that strategies for AIDS prevention have drawn on the lessons learned from family planning. In fact, just like early family planning programs, AIDS prevention has focused on women, at times to the exclusion of men. (Campbell 1995, 206)

However, the way men have been reached in these endeavors indeed parallels the way they have been reached within the field of HIV/AIDS prevention. Three tactics have been attempted in the area of reproductive health. The first tends to focus on the reproductive health problems caused by a system of gender inequality wherein men are more powerful and women are more powerless (and wherein men's beliefs about women and their resultant social practices are viewed as harming women). This approach leads to a gendered power and "women's empowerment" model (detailed in chapter 3). The second approach reaches out to men as "partners" in reproductive health and focuses on men helping women to achieve women's own reproductive goals. The approach says little about working with men to focus on their own health needs and assumes that men should work to improve women's health. Little is said about the ways in which race and class relations might inflect gendered approaches. However, numerous scholars have underscored the importance of working with men, and an example is stated by Pulerwitz and colleagues in 2010 when they argued that "[i]n the mid-1990s, the International Conference on Population and Development in Cairo and the International Conference on Women in Beijing called global attention to the importance of involving men in reproductive health programs because of their influence on women's health, including women's ability to protect themselves from infection with the human immunodeficiency virus (HIV)" (Pulerwitz et al. 2010, 1). Finally, a third approach both views work with men as focused on improving women's reproductive health and recognizes men as having health needs of their own. This approach views men as

> members of a family, usually as husbands, with a significant locus of responsibility for reproduction. The framework, therefore, envisions male involvement in reproduction and addresses men's own bio-reproductive and psycho-sexual needs. . . . [The framework] emphasizes a client-based approach that seeks to provide sustainable reproductive health care for men without compromising (and hopefully improving) services for women. Such a perspective recognizes men's important contributions to reproductive health, as well as men's needs, and attempts to reconcile conflicting reproductive goals within the context of reproductive partnerships, primarily married couples. (Dudgeon & Inhorn 2004, 1382)

A framework that "involves" men can easily gloss over some key aspects of power relations between women and men because women and men may occupy different positions in the terrain of relationship negotiations and social institutions. It also doesn't recognize that informing men about women's needs may or may not lead them to be more responsive, given gender-based power differentials in relationships (Pulerwitz, Gortmaker, & DeJong 2000; Pulerwitz et al. 2002). All of these various approaches can be differentiated from a fourth and a fifth approach—an "intersectional" approach and a "gender-transformative" approach to masculinities, sexuality, and HIV prevention (examined in much more depth in chapters 3 and 4). Rather than viewing men solely as responsible for harms to women's health (and asking them to be more responsible for improving women's health) and rather than viewing men *only* as partners who need to work to improve women's health, gender-transformative programming works to challenge the narrow and constraining definitions of masculinity that shape men's and women's health, shifting men in the direction of gender equality in the name of improving their own and others' health.

Given the importance of gender relations to HIV prevention, it is also critical to define the world of evidence-based HIV prevention programs that will be referred to throughout this book. Public-health and global-health programs can be categorized as "gender-insensitive," "gender-neutral," "gender-sensitive," "gender-empowering," and "gender-transformative" (Gupta 2001). "Gender-insensitive programming" refers to interventions that are "defined as efforts fostering predatory, violent, irresponsible images of male sexuality and portray women as powerless victims or as repositories of infection" (Gupta 2001, 9). In contrast to gender-insensitive interventions, gender-neutral programs do not enact harm by putting forward these stereotypical images of gender, but these also do not take gender norms into account and "fail to distinguish between the unique needs and circumstances of women and men" in HIV prevention (Gupta 2001, 9). Gender-sensitive programs "recognize women's and men's differing needs and constraints" (Gupta 2001, 10) but may or may not to work to change gender norms that shape HIV risk. Gender-empowering interventions seek to "empower women or free women and men from the impact of destructive gender and sexual norms" (Gupta 2001, 10) and work through collective action.

Finally, gender-transformative interventions "seek to transfigure gender roles and create more gender equitable relationships" (Gupta 2001, 10). In chapter 4, I will evaluate the impact of a women's rights–based and masculinities-focused gender-transformative HIV-prevention and antiviolence intervention on gender relations, violence, and HIV-related sexual practices.

While the shift to gender-transformative HIV-prevention interventions for heterosexually active men is rather new in the global realm (the last seven years), for quite some time now, HIV-prevention interventions for women have been theoretically informed by gender-related theories (e.g., a structural theory of gender and power—El-Bassel et al. 2003; Wingood & Diclemente 2000, 2002) and have advanced from being gender neutral to being more gender sensitive and gender transformative (Exner et al. 2003; Gupta 2001). Gina Wingood and colleagues innovatively applied Raewyn Connell's theory of gender and power (Connell 1987) to the case of HIV/AIDS prevention approximately fifteen years ago, in 2000. In the years that followed, several rigorous HIV-prevention programs in the funded science base have deployed this theory or researchers have modified gender-neutral social-psychological models to be more gender specific (for a review of this transition, see Exner et al. 2003). All of these HIV-prevention programs have resulted in successful risk-reduction outcomes for women (DiClemente et al. 2004; Ehrhardt et al. 2000, 2002; El-Bassel et al. 2003; Wingood et al. 2004, 2011).

In contrast with the global science base, where HIV prevention work focused on masculinity and gender-transformative work exists and may be on the rise, there is barely any of this work that has been funded in the United States. In order to follow up on any new work that had been published after the previously mentioned reviews, I led a systematic review of HIV interventions with heterosexually active men that was published in *AIDS & Behavior* with Sheri Lippman and Sarah Treves-Kagan (2013). We found that only Tello et al. (2010), Rhodes et al. (2011), and Zuloski & Cupples (2008) had worked to reshape norms of masculinity to reduce HIV-risk behaviors with heterosexually active men in the United States. Two of these three programs are with Latino men, one program is with youth, and *none* of the programs are focused on the population of African American, heterosexually active, adult men. This is the case despite the fact that more than one in five incident (new) infections with Black men are transmitted through sex with women in the United States, according to the CDC. For these men, masculinities take on nuanced and important meanings (this will be fleshed out in chapter 2) because of the intersection of sexual intimacy and structural constraints whereby racism, unemployment, housing instability or lack of housing, poverty, and incarceration are commonly experienced (Adimora, Schoenbach, & Floris-Moore 2009; Bowleg & Raj 2012; Mackenzie 2013; Raj & Bowleg 2012). In the United States, prevention programs do not intervene on the basis of gender—or racial inequality, or structural inequalities—much for heterosexually active men, even for those men who are most affected by HIV. In the one available evidence-based HIV-prevention program at the Centers for Disease Control that does attempt to intervene with men who have recently been released from prison (project START, in which 52% of participants were African American, 13.8% were Hispanic, 23% were White, and 12% were "other"), none of the intervention materials are focused on gender or masculinity (Wolitski et al. 2006).

In the systematic reviews mentioned above, we found that few programs for heterosexually active men were focused on masculinity and that for those that could be deemed gender sensitive and/or gender transformative, no changes in gender or race relations were attempted at the structural or institutional level. Nearly all of the "transformation" was at the level of individualized gender roles. Wait!? "Transformation" is being offered at the level of gender roles in evidence-based HIV-prevention interventions in the United States and around the world? Wasn't "gender roles" a White, middle-class, 1950s–1970s concept in the United States that had a large number of limitations—and for decades received a litany of critiques from sociology, from other disciplines, and from other nations? A short meander through such sociological reminders is an important and necessary exercise for the interdisciplinary field of HIV prevention before we move on to the vulnerability paradigm that is used to explain heterosexually active women's and men's HIV risks in chapter 2

A Brief History of "Male Gender Roles" and "Masculine Ideology" and Its Application to HIV Prevention

From the 1950s to the 1980s, important contributions were made to systematically delineate components of the "male role" within the disciplines of psychology and sociology. One widely referenced frame-work from David and Brannon included four main aspects of the male role: "No Sissy Stuff," "Be a Big Wheel," "Be a Sturdy Oak," and "Give 'Em Hell" (1976). Along with the feminist movement of several waves, it is here where the idea that masculinity and femininity are socially constructed, harmful to both women and men, and malleable in culture was developed. In early work, psychologists such as Pleck (1981, 1983) drew on role theory from more of a "trait-based" perspective, examin-ing masculinity as a characteristic that men "have" and as partly derived psychoanalytically from young men's relationships with their mothers and fathers. Approximately ten years later, work shifted away from the "trait-based" perspective to draw on more of a constructionist per-spective, which saw masculinity not as a fixed trait that an individual possesses but rather as a normative conception of what men "should be" (and therefore aspire to in beliefs and practices) according to cultural or societal-level definitions. With the shift to an understanding of mascu-linity as a normative conception, the term "masculinity ideology" was then introduced in research. Several researchers have underscored the difficulties that men experienced when adhering to norms of individual-ism, competitiveness, and the need to win by noting an emotional and psychological impoverishment in private life (Pleck, Sonnestein, & Ku 1993). Contemporary scholars in the areas of sexual health and sexuality have taken an interest in the paradox of men being and feeling powerful while also fearing feelings of vulnerability, thereby revealing the com-plexities of juggling between masculine ideals of conquest and desires for emotional intimacy and love (Brod 1988, 1995; Seal, Wagner-Raphael, & Ehrhardt 2000; Seal & Ehrhardt 2003).

Researchers interested largely in women's vulnerability to HIV/AIDS have examined the link between either male gender roles, male gen-der norms, or "traditional masculine ideologies" and HIV/AIDS. Here, men are deemed to have greater decision-making or absolute power in the initiation, pace, and orchestration of sexual activity and safer sex decisions (Amaro 1995; Byers 1996; Campbell, 1995; Exner et al. 1999; O'Sullivan & Byers 1992; Rutter & Schwartz 2011). Furthermore, narrow cultural definitions of masculinity can normalize sex as a competitive win when there is an assumption of a right to bodily access and pleasure from multiple women's bodies in the sexual double standard (Barker

2000; Exner et al. 2003; Campbell 1999; Gupta 2001; Logan, Cole, & Leukefeld 2002; Seal & Ehrhardt 2003). Additionally, norms of adventure, risk taking, and sexual conquest can meld together to constitute masculinity in ways that increase risky or coercive sexual behavior, particularly in male-dominated institutions such as sporting organizations, military establishments, bars, and fraternities (Bowleg et al. 2011; Crosset, Benedict, & McDonald 1995; Crosset 2000; Curry 1991; Pleck, Sonenstein, & Ku 1993; Messner & Stevens 2002). In short, "male gender roles" as these are socialized, masculinity as an ideological belief system that is structurally supported, and structural inequities in gendered power are seen to influence risky sexual behaviors that affect both men and women. Despite the fact that HIV researchers have drawn upon a mix of conceptual views on masculinity (as a gender role, as a gender norm, and as an ideology that men adhere to that influences their behaviors), HIV prevention has largely interpreted "masculinity" and "gender relations" in terms of a socialized role or norm and not a structurally supported set of institutions and practices nor as a collective practice (which is a central aspect of how sociologists view gender relations).

Within sociology, Stacey & Thorne (1985), Connell (1987, 1995a), Messner (1997), and others have put forward several criticisms of role theory, but these have not frequently found their way into HIV/AIDS-prevention interventions. Role theory has been critiqued for tending to rely on individualistic concerns about gendered beliefs and attitudes while negating structural and institutional analyses of power (Messner 1997; Stacey & Thorne 1985). This type of emphasis has also been criticized for being influenced by Talcott Parsons's sense of male and female roles within functionalist modes of social theory—instrumentality for men and expressiveness for women (Parsons & Bales 1955). The notion of roles in this framework is said to "retain its functionalist roots, emphasizing consensus, stability, and continuity. The notion of 'role' focuses more on individuals than social structure, and implies that 'the female role' and the 'male role' are complementary. The terms are depoliticizing; they strip experience from its historical and political context and neglect questions of power and conflict" (Stacey & Thorne 1985, 307).

A focus on roles has also tended to pin the need for social change on women, requiring them to change themselves without parallel attention being paid to targeting men (Campbell 1995). Additionally, feminist researchers have been wary of simply adding men to a role analysis, given that this can result in a simplified conclusion that men and women are "equally oppressed" by gender norms and can thereby sideline an analysis of gender inequality and the way it affects women. Put another way, focusing on roles is also critiqued for examining the problematic aspects of male gender norms such as "costs to masculinity" (that will be examined throughout this book) without offering simultaneous analytical weight to subjects of institutional inequalities (structural-level power) and the privileges associated with masculinity, or inequalities among different groups of men (Messner 1997).

In some ways, recognition of gender roles and norms among men in the HIV epidemic at least moved the field forward by recognizing the dynamic interplay of gendered social interactions and moved towards an understanding that gender is accomplished or done (West & Zimmerman 1987; West & Fenstermaker 1995). In other ways, this analytical move seemed to uncritically pin together the parts of the sex-gender-sexuality triad, assuming that people who were born male would socially enact *one* gender role in sex (that of hegemonic masculinity) and that this was naturally linked to heterosexuality within sexual intimacy. Furthermore, if within the field of HIV prevention the prescription for reducing HIV rates is that gender should just be "done differently" by individuals, then there is the need to also recognize the structural/institutional and historically patterned nature of gender and race relations and the flaws of "just do it" approaches to gender (Dworkin & Messner 1999). These approaches have failed to adequately engage with sociological concepts of agency and constraint beyond the individual level.

In Courtenay's crucial work, which provides a theory of the link between masculinity and poor health that looks beyond roles (i.e., adds to earlier conceptualizations of masculinity and poor health that underscored that "masculinity is hazardous to your health!" [Harrison, Chin, & Ficarotto 1995]), he argues that

> [m]en do not [act as they do] because of their role identities or psychological traits, but because of concepts about femininity and masculinity that they adopt from their culture. Gender is not two static categories, but rather "a set of socially constructed relationships which are produced and reproduced through people's actions" [Gerson & Peiss 1985]; it is con-

structed by dynamic, dialectic relationships. Gender is "something that one does, and does recurrently, in interaction with others" [West & Zimmerman 1987, 140]; it is achieved or demonstrated and is better understood as a verb than as a noun. Most importantly, gender does not reside in the person, but rather in social transactions defined as gendered. From this perspective, gender is viewed as a dynamic social structure. (2000b, 1387)

Thus, while it has been critical to move towards an analysis of masculinity in HIV prevention, the focus has mainly been on "male roles" and "male norms" that can be modified at the individual level. Still, I want to be clear that bolstering an analysis of male norms and roles within the field of HIV/AIDS prevention could lead to a solid push for more gender-equitable relationships and better health in a variety of ways. First, an analysis of roles for men within the epidemic is important because researchers have found that health-seeking behaviors (or their avoidance) are constitutive of masculine identities (Courtenay 2000a, 2000b). In this case, lack of health-seeking behaviors may help to bolster masculine identity and is played out by men to avoid perceptions of weakness, to bolster perceptions of independence, self-reliance, strength, and respect, or "to exert power and produce effects in their lives" (Courtenay 2000a).

Second, the social practices that men enact that undermine their own and women's health are often the instruments that men use in the maintenance and acquisition of masculinity, particularly if men do not have the structural means to attain masculinity because of structural inequalities (bolstering masculinity in these circumstances may mean multiple partners, risky adventure, dismissal of the need for help, sexual conquest, or violence against women or men) (Courtenay 2000b). Third, separating sex from gender and considering masculinity as a role linked to sex that is not wholly immersed in the natural realm would certainly allow for an uncoupling of sex from gender in the sex-gender-sexuality triad. This would allow a shift away from biological reductionism (as expressed, for example, in assumptions that men naturally need more sex, assumptions that men want sex all the time, assumptions that men cannot control their desire, or assumptions that men need women to say yes to sex or else they are being denied an essential need or demand) and a move toward an analysis of social expectations as differentially shaping women's and men's behaviors.

Fourth, challenging gender norms and roles offers a clear politics of health reform (fewer sexual partners, less violence, etc.) through changed expectations and understandings by individuals, groups, and organizations. And fifth, given the relationship among masculinity, violence, sexual relationship power, and women's HIV/AIDS risks (Dunkle et al. 2006; Jewkes, Dunkle, et al. 2006; Peacock & Levack 2004; Pulerwitz et al. 2002), reconstructing masculine norms to challenge the current gender order could also be a crucial step in (re)shaping gender equality and combating the global epidemic.

Ultimately, however, it is critical to consider what the impact is when HIV-prevention researchers include men in prevention programs without providing a theoretical frame that examines masculinities. If masculinities are not taken into account in HIV programs, then men are assumed to (a) not have gender (Kimmel 1990); (b) experience HIV risks that are not related to gender relations and gender inequality (i.e., are assumed to be at risk only on the basis of race, class, or sexuality marginalization and not on the basis of gender or the intersection of these factors); (c) be harmful to women (here, researchers are not considering how gender inequality structures both women's and men's HIV risks); (d) be a homogeneous group, an assumption that negates the reality that some men pay more dearly for being constrained to adhere to narrow definitions of masculinity than do others (Messner 1997; Sabo & Gordon 1995); and (e) not experience disjunctures between sexual identity and sexual acts, an assumption that misses the fact that these disjunctures can hinge on expressions of masculinity, particularly within groups of race- and class-marginalized men (Malebranche et al. 2009) (this will be explored in chapter 2, although the term "disjuncture" itself shows an overreliance on fixed categories). Merely providing men with information and skills within prevention programs—and predicting that they will enact changed behaviors once they receive these—negates that race and gender relations profoundly shape men's enactment of "risky behaviors" (Courtenay 2000a, 2000b; Kimmel 1990; Sabo & Gordon 1995). As has been highlighted by Courtenay (2000b),

> The consistent, underlying presumption in medical literature is that what it means to be a man in America has no bearing on how men work, drink, drive, fight, or take risks. Even in studies that address health risks more

common to men than women, the discussion of men's greater risks and of the influence of men's gender is often conspicuously absent. (1387)

The research offered in the HIV/AIDS-prevention science base, particularly in intervention work, tends to assume that gender is something that is easily done and undone once individuals are offered some information or encouragement as to how to do it differently. This assumption, paradoxically, asks researchers to face some of the same challenges raised earlier in the epidemic surrounding erroneous assumptions of rational choice and agency in individual-level theories in the early HIV/AIDS-prevention days. That is, public health mainly tends to recognize gendered, racialized, and classed power relations as part of the context that impacts HIV risk, but then tends to emphasize measures for behavioral change that suggest that women or men only need to agentically draw on their individual ability to "do" their sexual socialization differently.

The same debate (about whether one can simply do and undo gender) rages across disciplines, where an emphasis on negotiating certain gender roles or on "doing gender" as an "accomplishment" in an interactionist manner (West & Zimmerman 1987; West & Fenstermaker 1995) can be critiqued as a step away from the limitations of static gender roles, but also as failing to truly take the gendered, racialized, classed nature of power relations into account (Stacey & Thorne 1985; West & Fenstermaker 1995). Despite the more "active" stance implied by "doing gender," which may be an improvement over "gender roles," some of the same limitations are alive and well in both sets of concepts.

Changing gender roles and norms has been and will continue to be vital for HIV research, but can surely be further developed. First, it is important to understand the historical impetus for a call to change gender roles and norms. One main assumption of "choice" and "freedom" underlying liberal feminist thought was that if men and women could toss off restrictive roles, then this would be a move towards an egalitarian society (Friedan 1964; Dworkin & Messner 1999). Restrictive or "harmful" aspects of gender roles have long been viewed as part of what is called a liberal feminist stance within the United States, and has been translated into public-health and global-health interventions as the "sociocultural context" of gender norms. But similarly to any call for

changes to women surrounding gender norms, this leaves the most privileged and/or efficacious women (or the most egalitarian men) facing
the greatest possibilities for enacting "success," all too frequently negating the range of complexities faced by the more constrained (Dworkin
& Messner 1999; Messner 2002; Heywood & Dworkin 2003). For men,
there are precisely parallel and similar challenges that need to be considered (below and in chapters 2, 4, and 5).

In 2009 in an article in the *American Journal of Public Health*,
Fullilove, Peacock, and I underscored that the point made above is
particularly important for HIV/AIDS scholars in the case of economically disadvantaged men who may be race and/or class oppressed, and
are frequently kept from traditional definitions of masculine success
(high-paying jobs, freedom from police harassment, freedom from
imprisonment, or access to jobs to begin with). Put another way, what
some scholars call "the signifiers of 'true' masculinity (e.g., sexual conquest, physical forms of masculinity) are readily accessible to men who
may otherwise have limited resources for constructing masculinity"
(Courtenay 2000b, 1392). What this means is that marginalized men
may therefore be more reliant on enacting narrow definitions of hegemonic masculinity in sex as a means of constructing masculine status
(Majors & Billson 1992; Messner 1997) in societal terms where men
are denied structural opportunities to be "real men" (i.e., hegemonic
men). Thus, sexual intimacy can play an important role for men in the
social constitution of masculinity. For these men, critical reflections
on the role of masculinity in shaping both men's and women's health
and sexuality are crucial.

Overall, then, assuming that information alone can help men to
avoid HIV/AIDS risks (e.g., information on the importance of using
condoms and on how to use a condom) and assuming that they will
modify gender-related behaviors negates the reality that race, class, and
gender relations profoundly shape men's agency (Courtenay 2000a,
2000b; Kimmel 1990; Sabo & Gordon 1995) in sexual practices. An
emphasis on masculinity and gender relations would move HIV prevention in the United States further in the direction where key masculinity scholars in the United States and worldwide have progressed
for decades and where public-health and global-health scholars have
shifted more recently (Barker et al. 2007, 2010; Peacock & Levack 2004;

Pulerwitz, Michaelis et al. 2010; Raj et al. 2013; Verma et al. 2008). But before we examine the promises and limitations of HIV-prevention interventions that focus solely on gendered power and "women's empowerment" (leaving heterosexually active men out) or examine the promises and limitations of gender-transformative health interventions with heterosexually active men, we first need to determine whether heterosexually active men are indeed "vulnerable" to HIV/AIDS. That is the subject of the next chapter.

2

Vulnerable Women, Invulnerable Men?

The Need for Intersectionality in HIV/AIDS Prevention

Even though over twenty thousand women in the United States had cumulatively died of AIDS by the end of 1992, they were not officially counted as AIDS victims. Unfortunately, the early AIDS case definition used by the Centers for Disease Control (CDC) left women out entirely: it did not include several disease manifestations that were common to women, including invasive cervical cancer and recurrent vaginal yeast infections (CDC 1992; Hankins and Handley 1992; Higgins, Hoffman, & Dworkin 2010; Wright et al. 1994), and hence women were not being counted as having AIDS. Soon, greater clinical understanding that women's recurrent yeast infections were opportunistic infections indicative of AIDS was achieved. Forces to change the official AIDS case definition came from outrage at the mass deaths, legal pressures, activism and advocacy from women's groups (and their intersection), and a resounding wealth of international data. And at long last, the AIDS case definition was formally expanded in 1993 to include the disease manifestations described above that were common indicators of AIDS in women (CDC 1992). Women could then be counted.

Only then could she arrive, be breathed into existence, surface into the light of day: the "vulnerable" heterosexual woman. Newfound visibility was crucial on the public health front for women in terms of HIV/AIDS prevention, treatment, and care. It meant that women might be less likely to be excluded from drug trials and from studies of disease progression than they had been in the past (Berer 1993; Fox-Tierney et al. 1999; Strebel 1995). It meant that women with access to health care might be less likely to receive inadequate diagnoses, to have a poor understanding of disease manifestation, or to experience delayed treatment (Amaro, Raj, & Reed 2001; Cohan & Atwood 1994). At the juncture of shifting surveillance categories was a continually moving base of medical knowledge alongside of epidemiological classifications, advocacy, sexual stratification systems, and the gendered discursive realm—the result was that women were increasingly counted, and their attendant needs for care and prevention made more possible.

But within and across categories, the issue of who becomes "epidemiologically fathomable" (an earlier version of this framework appears in Dworkin 2005)—that is, who is counted, who is left out, and the attendant discourses of vulnerability that circulate through the public around these categories—leaves us all with much to critically untangle. In this chapter, I first critically examine the widely offered statement that women are regarded as especially vulnerable to HIV/AIDS in the United States and worldwide. I focus on HIV transmission among women and men of different races, sexualities, or regions. I seek to examine the epidemiology and social nature of vulnerability and to question overdetermined notions of vulnerable women and invulnerable men that rely on certain assumptions about gender relations and certain specific singular linkages in a sex-gender-sexuality triad.

First, I examine and challenge the underlying emphasis in public health discourse on the popular frame of "vulnerable women" who acquire HIV through "heterosexual transmission." Drawing on the insights of epidemiologists, HIV/AIDS scholars, and theories that both draw upon and challenge monolithic understandings of a sex-gender-sexuality triad (multiracial feminist intersectionality in particular), I reintroduce the question of why a discourse of vulnerability is so thoroughly infused into the issue of women's but not men's heterosexual transmission and "risk." I also examine a framework of intersectionality, examine how this has been used in the literature outside of HIV/AIDS, and address how, even though it clearly applies to the epidemiology of HIV/AIDS, such a framework does not structure evidence-based prevention interventions with women and men. Finally, I briefly examine the hierarchical classification system that is used to label HIV acquisition for women and men in the HIV epidemic. Here, I critically underscore the way in which singular, hierarchical surveillance categories help to constitute the emergence of the "high-risk" and "vulnerable" heterosexual woman who is implied by the heterosexual transmission category while simultaneously constituting the failure to fathom heterosexually active men's, bisexual men's, and lesbian and bisexual women's transmission risk (and women as agents overall). In the final portion of the chapter, I make suggestions for to how to push beyond current "gendered" or "sexualized" understandings of which women and men are epidemiologically fathomable and therefore vulnerable in terms of HIV transmission (Albert 2001; Dowsett 1996, 2002, 2003; Connell & Dowsett 1999; Higgins, Hoffman, & Dworkin 2010; Morrow & Allsworth 2000; Reeves 2003).

The (Gendered) Heterosexual Couple? Vulnerable Women, Invulnerable Men?

In 1994, heterosexual transmission surpassed intravenous drug use as the predominant route of transmission to U.S. women with a diagnosis of AIDS (CDC 1995). This is now the largest category of identifiable risk in women (CDC 2013e). Indeed, in the initial surveillance categories in the early to mid-1990s, heterosexual contact was said to constitute 60% of the identifiable HIV risk for women, and in 2013, this number had risen to 86% (CDC, 2013e). Women now account for nearly one in five new HIV infections in the United States (CDC 2013b). And, from 1987 to 2009, the percentage of women among persons who died from HIV infection increased from 10% to 28% (CDC 2011).

Within the HIV literature, women are frequently deemed "more" or "especially" vulnerable to HIV infection in comparison to men due to a combination of biological and social susceptibility factors. In terms of biological factors, it is suggested that women are exposed to infectious fluids for longer periods of time during sexual intercourse than men are; they are said to have an increased risk of tissue injury during intercourse; and in the genital tracts of young women, cervical mucous is more penetrable and the squamocolumnar junction is situated on the surface of the cervix, exposing a greater proportion of columnar epithelium, a target site for HIV (Kaiser Family Foundation 2012a; MacPhail, Williams, & Campbell 2002; Padian et al., 1997; Royce et al. 1997; UNAIDS 2012). Due to genital physiology, then, and the nature and pattern of sexual relationships, studies generally cite that male-to-female transmissibility is about twice that of female-to-male transmission (Campbell 1995, 1999; CDC 2011; Logan, Cole, & Leukefeld 2002; MacPhail, Williams, & Campbell 2002; Padian et al. 1997). The claim of women being twice as likely as men to acquire HIV is "strengthened by analogy with other (albeit bacterial) sexually transmitted infections such as chlamydia and gonorrhea," which also exhibit "different transmission probabilities from men to women than from women to men" (Moench et al. 2001 as cited in Higgins, Hoffman, & Dworkin 2010, 436).

The HIV literature does not suggest that biological "vulnerability" is the only set of susceptibility factors that make women "especially vulnerable" to the disease. As was mentioned in chapter 1, there are also a large number of social factors that are commonly identified as leading to women's greater vulnerability to HIV in comparison to men's. Here, scholars argue that women's economic and social subordination to men is coupled with a sexual double standard that condones men's nonmonogamy while expecting monogamy from women (Exner et. al. 2003; Gómez & VanOss Marin 1996; Gupta 2001, 2002). Unequal economic and social status has been found to put women at a distinct disadvantage in terms of gendered power relations and negotiating sexual encounters (Exner et al. 2003; Grieg & Koopman 2003; Preston-Whyte et al. 2000).

Other research that examines the social vulnerabilities that shape HIV risks has found that food insecurity is associated (both domestically and globally) with greater HIV/AIDS vulnerabilities (though the exchange of food for sex) for women but not for men (Anema et al. 2009; Tsai, Hung, & Weiser 2012; Weiser et al. 2007). And, marriage itself has been mentioned earlier as a major risk factor for women globally. Aside from research showing that this may be due to women erroneously assuming that their primary partnership is safe (in a sexual double standard where they may be monogamous while their partner is not), some argue that this has to do with a gendered opportunity structure that differentiates access to the public versus private sphere for women versus men, coupled with gendered divisions of labor within these realms (Hirsch et al. 2002).

In addition to examining structural factors, some researchers draw more implicitly or explicitly on ideas about gender socialization and/ or psychoanalytic theories to argue that women are relationally defined, socialized to put their needs aside in the interest of pleasing others (Amaro 1995; Amaro, Raj, & Reed 2001; Chodorow 1978; Maxwell & Boyle 1995; Exner, Seal, & Ehrhardt 1997; Reid 2000). This "other-orientedness," coupled with a desire to sustain relationships, inequitable gendered power relations, and a broader discourse that privileges male pleasure in sex, leads many HIV researchers to put forth that men and women tend to make a male partner's sexual pleasure central, increasing risks to women (Amaro 1995; Amaro, Raj, & Reed 2001; Exner et al. 2003; Reid 2000; Sobo 1995). It is also argued that other risks for heterosexually active women are women's "passive" orientation to knowing their own bodies or sexual needs and beliefs that women should not have sexual knowledge given the constraints set out in the madonna/whore dichotomy—this too can keep women from asserting their needs or more actively participating in condom decisions (Blumstein & Schwartz 1983; Byers 1996; O'Sullivan & Byers 1992; Ortiz-Torres, Williams, & Ehrhardt 2003; Rutter & Schwartz 2011). Even if women can negotiate actively for condom use, many women do not, putting them most "at risk" with their current long-term male partner, because desires for trust, intimacy, and pleasure can lead to the (erroneous) assumption that a primary sexual relationship is safe (Ehrhardt et al. 1992; Hirsch et al. 2007, 2010; Simoni, Walters & Nero 2000; Exner et al. 2003).

In addition, research shows that structural and interpersonal dimensions between women and men intersect to produce women's vulnerability to HIV—researchers who have quantitatively measured women's relationship power (SRPS—the Sexual Relationship Power Scale) find that women with lower relationship power have a harder time negotiating safe sex with their partners (Pulerwitz, Gortmaker, & DeJong 2000; Pulerwitz et al. 2002). The Sexual Relationship Power Scale has been a groundbreaking way to characterize unequal relationships between women and men in heterosexually active relationships and is constituted by a "decision-making dominance" subscale and by a "relationship control" subscale—both of which have been found to be associated with women's HIV risks. That is, the more control that men exert in relationships with women—and the more decision-making dominance that men have relative to women—the more women are likely to face barriers to active condom-use decision making. While studies such as these began in the United States among Latina women, this finding has been replicated in other countries and populations, such as in South Africa among women attending antenatal care clinics. In the South African study, researchers find that high levels of male control in relationships are associated with HIV seropositivity, and the authors "postulate that abusive men are more likely to have HIV and impose risky sexual practices on partners" (Dunkle et al. 2004, 1415).

Violence and the fear of violence are also recognized as important risk factors contributing to the vulnerability to HIV infection for women. Violence and fear of abandonment act as significant barriers to condom use for women, who have to negotiate use of condoms, communicate about fidelity with their partners, or leave relationships that they perceive as risky (Dunkle et al. 2004; Lang et al. 2013; Weiss & Gupta 1998). Research from around the world now consistently shows that women who experienced physical and sexual abuse from their husbands were several times more likely to become infected with HIV than women who were not abused (Jewkes, Dunkle et al. 2006, 2010; Jewkes et al. 2011; Shi, Kouyoumdjian, & Dushoff 2013; Silverman et al. 2008). Research in the United States that was drawn from the National Epidemiological Survey on Alcohol and Related Conditions and analyzed 13,928 women found that women who experience violence from their partners were more than three times as likely to have HIV infection as women who do not. In one study, almost 12% of HIV infection among women was found to be due to intimate partner violence (Sareen, Pruga, & Grant 2009).

Several studies at the University of California at San Francisco confirm the link between HIV risk and physical and psychological abuse. For example, Machtinger et al. (2012a) carried out a meta-analysis of previous studies examining rates of psychological trauma and PTSD among HIV-positive women in the United States. They found that HIV-positive women have experienced PTSD at a rate —30%—that is five times higher than that of women in the general population. In this study, they also found that 55% of women who were HIV positive experienced intimate partner violence, which is twice the national rate of violence against women. Finally, in another 2012 study (Machtinger et al. 2012b), the same team examined data from a prevention program with HIV-positive women and transgender women and found that those with recent trauma had three times the odds of reporting unsafe sex with a partner and four times the odds of nonadherence to their antiretroviral therapy than did those who had not experienced trauma.

There are other structural inequalities that intersect with social practices that can make women "vulnerable" to HIV acquisition. For example, in my own collaborative research that was carried out with the Kenyan Medical Research Institute (KEMRI) and GROOTS-Kenya (Grassroots Women Organizing Together in Kenya—a network of women's community-based organizations and self-help groups that work to empower women locally), I examined how women's lack of property rights in southern and eastern Africa contributes to their HIV risks. In the research project that I led in Nyanza and Western Provinces, Kenya (where HIV rates are 25–33% and property rights violations are common), I found (and this has been found elsewhere) that when husbands died of HIV and AIDS, women were often blamed for the illness (even if they did not bring HIV into the household) and were subsequently thrown out of the their homes (disinherited). But the women were not simply disinherited. The in-laws frequently carried out "property grabbing" (stealing her property—even though she is the next of kin on the title) and "asset stripping" (taking all of her belongings, including livestock, pots, pans, clothing, and more) right when the woman was grieving the death of her husband.

Thus, when women were disinherited, they were thrown out of their homes with no belongings, nowhere to go, and no social networks. To survive, women migrated to new settings to look for shelter and work, often with their children—settings where they experienced high levels of sexual risk due to poverty and the exchange of sex for shelter, food, and clothing, or due to their taking on an increased number of partners in order to make ends meet (Camlin, Kwena, & Dworkin 2013; Dworkin, Grabe et al. 2013; Lu et al. 2013). The HIV literature also reveals that widow inheritance (the practice of a widow whose husband has died of HIV/AIDS being "inherited" by the family, having sex with a male relative in order to be retained in the family), forced marriage, early marriage, the resurgence of temporary marriages, and, in certain circumstances, polygamy can increase women's and girls' HIV risks (Cheemeh et al. 2006; Obermeyer 2006; Lotfi et al. 2013).

It is suggested that all of the above "gendered" forces—economic, psychoanalytic, structural, interpersonal, social, and sociocultural—leave heterosexually active women hurt, disadvantaged, or erased in sexual encounters and in efforts to ensure sexual safety. Furthermore, in terms of actual numbers, heterosexual transmission as a risk category currently makes up a much larger proportion of women's risk compared to men's in the United States (CDC 2013e). Among men diagnosed with HIV infection, 81% are categorized as being infected from male-to-male sexual contact, 10% from sex with a woman, 5% from intravenous drug use, and 3% from a combination of drug use and male-to-male sexual contact (CDC 2013a). Among women diagnosed with HIV, 86% are said to have been infected through sex with a man, 13% from intravenous drug use, and less than 1% from "other" risks (CDC 2013a). But in terms of heterosexually active women and men, the question still remains as to why sexuality (heterosexuality) is only gendered in one particular way in attempts to explain women's vulnerability to HIV? How, after decades and decades of interdisciplinary challenges to singular notions of "sex" and "gender" and "sexuality" that feature passive, powerless, vulnerable emphasized femininity and aggressive, powerful, violent hegemonic masculinity could this still be one of the central narratives explaining women's HIV acquisition in the gender order (Connell 1987, 1995a)?

In 2010, Jenny Higgins, Susie Hoffman, and I underscored the advantages of the "vulnerability paradigm" (to be clear, we critique the language even as we drew upon it) in an article in the *American Journal of Public Health*. We described the importance of the term "vulnerability," as it clearly marked a critical transition from individual-level frameworks to those that include relational and structural factors that shape HIV risks. We also underscored that "recognition of women's structural disadvantage has been one of the vulnerability paradigm's most powerful and lasting contributions" (Higgins, Hoffman, & Dworkin 2010, 436). We stated that there was a paradox because the international community's response to a vulnerability paradigm was large and ushered in much-needed funding, policies, and programs for women's HIV risks but sometimes did so in racist ways that feature the vulnerability of "poor" women who need to be "saved," in a manner similar to the way "trafficked" women (or sex workers) are viewed as needing to be "saved" under conservative ideologies that aren't accurate or helpful in terms of respecting and recognizing human agency (Bernstein 2010; Lerum 1999; Kempadoo, Sanghera, & Pattanaik 2011). We also highlighted the powerful and important impacts that a vulnerability framework has had because it led to the development of gender-sensitive and gender-empowering HIV/AIDS-prevention programs that, as I pointed out in chapter 1, have shown tremendous success and efficacy in terms of reducing women's risk of HIV (DiClemente et al.

2004; Ehrhardt et al. 2000, 2002; El-Bassel et al. 2003; Miller et al. 2000; Wingood et al. 2004).

At the same time that the current paradigm has served important purposes and will continue to do so, it is vital to consider how the transmission "facts" for heterosexually active women and men have intersected with a limited set of theoretical assumptions in a sex-gender-sexuality triad. That is, within this paradigm, one of the most common concepts used to explain risk is that an analysis of the sex/gender system retains primacy over other analyses of "risk" and "vulnerability." Next, I will explain the sex/gender system that was introduced during the rise of first and second wave feminism and show how privileging the primacy of it has in fact prevented a more comprehensive analysis of intersectionality that is required before we can understand—and intervene upon—both women's and men's actual risks.

As I argued in my 1995 article in *Culture, Health, and Sexuality*, the notion of a sex/gender system was (re)introduced during the rise of second wave feminism by Gayle Rubin (1975) in her classic piece "The Traffic of Women." I don't raise Rubin's work to single out and criticize it—I raise this work as emblematic of a particular era of thinking (that Rubin herself has moved beyond) and in order to explain the sex/gender system as it has been taken up by HIV/AIDS scholars. In this work, heterosexuality was conceptualized as a specifically gendered and unequal material and social arrangement. The basis for women's oppression, Rubin argued, is the transformation of biological needs (sex) into a system of social relations (gender) through the kinship system. In such a system, women are transacted as gifts in the institution of marriage and it is the exchange partners, men, who are the beneficiaries of the exchange (heterosexuality). This exchange of women, she argues, is a means through which men are able to establish their dominance over women and constrain women's sexuality into being responsive to men's needs. Furthermore, the sexual division of labor, or the fact that women and men carry out separate tasks that receive widely varying cultural valuations, acts against male and female sameness, fuels gender inequality, and makes it economically difficult for women to achieve independence on their own without heterosexual relations.

As one can see, the sex/gender system as it was conceived at that time (decades ago) was drawn upon by HIV researchers, and this paradigm made certain assumptions about the linkages within the sex-gender-sexuality triad. The first main assumption within the sex/gender system that was brought into HIV studies was that heterosexual women are categorically oppressed/vulnerable while heterosexual men are categorically powerful/invulnerable. Second, there is the assumption that biological women have one gender role known as femininity (and are hurt by it in the HIV epidemic), while biological men have one gender role known as masculinity (and tend to hurt women with it) (both men and women are assumed to be 100% heterosexual). The third assumption that was brought into HIV studies from very early social science conceptions of gender is that the primacy of the sex-gender system in a sex-gender-sexuality triad can explain HIV risk over and above (or without) examining the intersection of race, class, gender, sexuality, or other social axes that may shape HIV risk.

To challenge a "discourse of vulnerability," my colleagues and I (Higgins, Hoffman, & Dworkin 2010) examined the literature assessing the state of the HIV/AIDS epidemic in various parts of the world. We found that the vulnerability paradigm is viewed as "true" even in places where it should have far less footing according to the epidemiology of HIV in that locale. In that paper, my colleague Susie Hoffman in particular wrote about how in some regions of the world where there are more generalized epidemics, such as eastern and southern Africa, women have always made up around 40–50% of the AIDS cases (Hankins & Hadley 1992). Earlier in the epidemic, we described how women were being infected by men who were thought to bring HIV into the relationship by a pattern of outside relationships (Anderson et al. 1991). Additionally, migration for work was also viewed as playing a role in exacerbating women's infections given that men who drove trucks or migrated were viewed as bridging populations by coming home and infecting their partners (Ramjee & Gouws 2002; Lurie 2000; Lurie et al., "The Impact" 2003; Lurie et al., "Who Infects Women?" 2003). Finally, current and past population-based surveys found that men are much more likely to be unfaithful to a primary partner than women are (Carael 1995; de Walque 2006; Nnko et al. 2004).

However, we argued that it is now much more plausible to suggest that another dynamic is playing a large role in sustaining the high HIV prevalence in generalized epidemics, and that is concurrency—or patterns of both partners having long-term simultaneous relationships (Epstein 2008; Halperin & Epstein 2004). In fact, several studies have suggested that patterns of concurrent long-term relationships may be a very powerful way to spread HIV (Garnett & Johnson 1997; Morris & Kretzschmar 1997; Watts & May 1992). Rapid infection can occur since social networks are densely connected, and where there is acute infection (an early point in a person's infectiousness when the person is highly infectious), HIV can be spread much more easily in this window. Furthermore, scholars are simply used to using the "male migrant model," and new research has underscored how female migrants and not simply male migrants have, at times, been the individuals who leave for work and return home, some of them returning HIV positive to infect their HIV-negative male partners (Lurie et al., "Who Infects Women?" 2003). And of course poverty itself can lead women to take on additional partners both domestically and globally in order to exchange sex for food, clothing, housing, or goods.

In that paper, we specifically noted why these assumptions matter for the HIV/AIDS epidemic and how researchers intervene on women's and men's risks:

> Large-scale heterosexual concurrent partnership networks cannot emerge or persist unless some women, in addition to men, have concurrent partners. Emerging data show that in many settings women are almost as likely as men to bring HIV into the partnership. An analysis of nationally representative demographic and health survey samples for Burkina Faso, Cameroon, Ghana, Kenya, and Tanzania found that in 30% to 40% of couples with 1 or both partners infected with HIV, the woman was positive and the man negative, even though relatively few women reported having outside partners (de Walque, 2006). In the Rakai district of Uganda, HIV+ women constitute a substantial proportion of serodiscordant couples (Serwadda et al., 1995), and in a study of migrant and non-migrant couples in rural South Africa, the woman was the infected partner in nearly one-third of the discordant couples (Lurie et al., 2003). (Higgins, Hoffman, & Dworkin 2010, 439)

We argued that evidence demonstrates that just as men bring HIV into their partnerships by their prior relationships or by having concurrent partners, women, too, bring HIV into their partnerships. This doesn't mean that we shouldn't attend to gender inequality and women's susceptibility to HIV. It does mean that we should be "dismayed ... that the vulnerability model considers only heterosexual women to be vulnerable to and socially disadvantaged by the disease" (Higgins, Hoffman, & Dworkin 2010, 439).

Similar analyses are starting to be carried out in the United States. Dolwick-Grieb, Davey-Rothwell, & Latkin (2012) desired to understand concurrent sexual partnerships among urban African American women and found that concurrency was associated with forced sex, drug use, incarceration of self and partner, and concurrency of the male partner. Nunn et al. (2012) studied concurrent sexual partnerships among African American women in Philadelphia and found that structural factors shaped concurrency among African American women. These included dependence on partners financially, the male partners' dependence on women, and incarceration. As early as 2003–2004, Adimora et al. (2003, 2004) found that a significant portion of African Americans in North Carolina who had reported HIV infection reported having concurrent partners. Thus, the assumption of male-only concurrency is not only inaccurate domestically and globally but leaves out important ways in which race, class, and gender inequalities intersect to restructure social and sexual relationships and intimacy in ways that shape HIV risk (MacKenzie 2013).

Therefore, it seems that singular linkages about vulnerability within the sex-gender-sexuality triad are being assumed and deployed domestically and around the globe in interventions on heterosexually active women's and men's HIV risk no matter what the dynamics of the epidemic actually are. Omitting a discourse of heterosexually active men's vulnerability is even more alarming when one thinks epidemiologically in particular. That is, as has been noted by Susie Hoffman at the Columbia University HIV Center for Clinical and Behavioral Studies (Higgins, Hoffman, & Dworkin 2010), women cannot be put at risk via sexual transmission with a heterosexually active male partner unless that male partner is already infected and thus clearly vulnerable and at risk. It would be useful to therefore reconsider the powerful men/powerless women paradigm that is embedded into early understandings of gender relations—to think carefully about the social and structural risks at hand, and to proceed with a theoretical model that characterizes actual risks (such as intersectionality, which will be defined and covered below). This is what the rest of the chapter will focus on, along with more critical examination of the ways in which surveillance categories operate to produce expectations around gender and vulnerability.

Researchers interested in women's vulnerability to HIV/AIDS privilege the logic of the second wave feminist gender order not only when studying women, femininity, and HIV/AIDS but also when studying men, masculinity, and HIV/AIDS. As has been underscored in chapter 1, men are conceived of as masculine, aggressive, less concerned with partners' sexual needs than their own, and unable or unwilling to control their bodily needs amidst a hydraulic model of desire. Men are conceived of in the HIV literature as having inordinate power and needing multiple partners or are viewed as violent, and it therefore remains somewhat curious that the term "especially vulnerable" is not taken up more frequently in the "epidemic of signification" (Treichler 1999a, 1999b) for heterosexually active men. In the articles that do conceive of heterosexually active men as vulnerable to HIV and openly state as much, this vulnerability is often said to be due to the way "the unequal power balance in gender relations increases men's vulnerability to HIV infection despite—or rather because of—their greater power" (Gupta 2001, 7). Other scholars agree that "effective HIV interventions may require" that men receive "help" with controlling "their impulses to be violent, coercive, or promiscuous" (Campbell 1995, 137) (this kind of language can all too easily elide into racist and essentialized assertions about people of color that this book contests). Here, too, in the HIV-prevention science base, men's power or individual-level problematic behavior is viewed as the "cause" of their (and women's) "risk" and acquisition of HIV (and not the way their race, class, age, migratory status, prison status, level of poverty, homelessness, incarceration history, cultural context, or all of these shape the collective practice of masculinities).

In my 2005 work, I underscored that there are several reasons for the less frequent or thorough considerations of heterosexually active men's vulnerability, even as heterosexual activity constitutes the second largest category of transmission in the United States for men and the first globally. Homophobia towards gay, MSM, or bisexual men may be operating rather significantly, because if public discourse prevents the creation of a language of vulnerability for heterosexual men (as opposed to an assumed gay or bi male "infectiousness"), then the familiar definition of heterosexual masculinity as powerful and femininity as vulnerable is reinforced (Treichler 1999b). That is, perhaps the supposedly less vulnerable "us" (the "real" men, heterosexual masculinity) is inextricably intertwined with a profound "othering" (the "fragile anus," the "promiscuous" MSM or bisexual, the sexual minority who "deserves" HIV) and contributes to the erasure of the vulnerability of all men (Patton 2002; Treichler 1999a, 1999b; Waldby 1996).

Another partial explanation for the lack of attention to heterosexually active men's vulnerability may be the way in which men are erroneously constituted as physically invulnerable within many societies. This should be questioned for numerous reasons, including the fact that many more men than women successfully commit suicide (Canetto 1995); die in wars (Connell 1995b; Fischer 2013; Kaufman 1994); are killed by other men on the streets (Harrison, Chin, & Ficarrotto 1995; Lozano et al. 2012); die from drinking and driving (Waldron 1995); die from steroid use (Klein 1993, 1995); experience devastating occupational hazards within male-dominated occupations (Courtenay 2000b; Harrison, Chin, & Ficarrotto 1995; Messner 1997, 2002); or die from HIV/ AIDS (UNAIDS 2012).

Another explanation for the lack of attention to heterosexually active men's vulnerability to HIV is the one that has been emphasized in this chapter—that men are conceived of as powerful in the gender order without recognition that they may be highly marginalized by race, class, and the disjuncture between sexual identities and sexual acts—and other social locations and contextual factors that profoundly shape masculinities and HIV/AIDS risks. This point will be thoroughly examined under the section on intersectionality and HIV/AIDS. And, there is also the possibility that because Black men are most affected by HIV in the United States, and Black men constitute by far the greatest number of men who are heterosexually infected—in the United States—and because much media fanfare has propagated the assumption that Black men acquire HIV from being on the "down low" (examined in this chapter), the reality of heterosexual transmission vulnerability "remains neglected in HIV program, policy, and research in the United States, despite growing epidemiologic data attesting to their needs" (Raj & Bowleg 2012, 179).

At this point, some readers might wonder how researchers dedicated to eradicating gender inequality or HIV risk due to gender relations would even begin to shift the limitations of current work, which often conceives of passive emphasized femininity and aggressive hegemonic masculinity as the key to inequality in a narrowly defined gender order (Dowsett 2003). Such questions have been consistently raised over the last several decades outside of HIV studies. Brief mention of some of these theorists raises vital challenges to research that privileges a particular relationship between gender and sexuality as "the" analytical angle in studies of HIV risk and vulnerability.

First, there has been much theoretical challenge offered to concepts of "gendered oppression" that conflate gender with women. Such concepts tend to rely on structuralist and modernist assumptions that power is categorically owned by men and is used to oppress and dominate women. These stances are flawed not only in terms of the assumption that "women" and "men" are unified or homogeneous categories but also for the ways in which power is conceived. These stances also do not take into account the fact of structural realities wherein disenfranchised women and men in many societies now face massive economic and social destabilization domestically and globally (Altman 2000; Lorber 1994, 1996; Plummer 2000). These forces and many others shape both women's and men's HIV risks.

Other challenges have been offered to the primacy-of-gender analysis (i.e., "women are more vulnerable") through not only queer theory and GLBT studies but also multiracial feminism, which has long argued that concepts of intersectionality (race, class, gender, and sexuality) may be more useful to any given analysis of identity, structural inequality, or day-to-day experience (Baca-Zinn & Thornton-Dill 1993; Eitzen & Baca-Zinn 1995; Hill-Collins 1986, 1990, 2005; Thornton-Dill 1988; Weeks 1985, 2002). Individuals do not have singular identities or experiences within social structures that expand or limit social practices, but rather, intersecting ones.

In the remaining portions of the chapter, then, I will introduce intersectionality as a concept and then show specifically why it matters for the HIV epidemic—and why prevention should draw upon it in its array of solutions. Intersectionality as a concept is credited to Kimberle Crenshaw, a critical race and legal scholar (1991). She drew much-needed attention to the ways in which legal scholars would focus on the most privileged aspects of various subordinated categories (e.g., whiteness is privileged in legal cases focused on gender, maleness is privileged in cases focused on race) when analyzing social injustices. She recognized that the "most marginalized" (in her analysis, Black women) can share qualities with dominant categories (e.g., Black men) while at the same time having unique experiences that are not captured within dominant categories drawn upon in legal cases (given the ways in which race, class, and gender intersect). Ultimately, she argued that the needs of African American women were left behind in the legal system because lawyers continually drew on case precedent that either privileged analyses of Blackness (without considering that African American women were also women—and these cases often focused on Black men) or privileged analyses of gender (without considering that Black women had needs not only as women but as African Americans—and these cases often focused on White women). Because of these limited theorizations that were applied to legal cases—that is, theorizations focusing either on gender or on race but not on their intersection—the needs of African American women were found to have fallen through the cracks in the legal system.

Numerous other scholars within multiracial feminism took up the study of intersectionality (Anzaldua, Cantu, & Hertado 2012; Baca-Zinn & Thornton-Dill 1993; Eitzen & Baca-Zinn 1995; Hill-Collins 1990, 1999; hooks 1984, 2000; Thornton-Dill 1988) for nearly three decades. Actually, such challenges to unitary conceptions of women have been alive and well for much longer, because we can count Sojourner Truth's brilliant narrative "Ain't I a Woman?" (1851) at the Women's Convention in Akron, Ohio, which challenged White men to consider that African American women were in fact women ("I have ploughed, and planted, and gathered into barns, and no man could head me! And ain't I a woman? I could work as much and eat as much as a man—when I could get it—and bear de lash as well! And ain't I a woman?"). It was not until 2004–2005 that HIV/AIDS studies began to take notice of frames of intersectionality. In 2004, Harvey and Bird started asking why studies of power only focused on a narrow conception of low relationship power, and in their qualitative work with African American women showed that women felt powerful when men stayed in relationships with them. This may be due to the way in which racism, deindustrialization, homicide, poverty, and the prison system interact to produce a greater ratio of women to men in the African American community.

The above material begins to point us to why intersectionality matters for HIV risks. This imbalanced sex ratio mentioned above has been found to exacerbate African American women's HIV risks in the United States and lead to less condom negotiating power (McNair & Prather 2004). Other scholars focused on the sex ratio underscore that "African-American women contending with the gender ratio imbalance that exists may relinquish negotiating power in their relationships, and may be more likely to settle for less desirable partners, accept infidelity, and agree to engage in unprotected sex" (Bowleg 2004, as cited in Newsome & Airhihenbuwa 2013, 461). Research has also found that men may be less likely to be responsive to women's requests to stop having other female partners because they know that there is a small pool of available African American men and that women will accept men having concurrent or multiple partners in order to have a partner (Thomas & Thomas 1999).

In 2005, Michelle Berger took up the idea of intersectionality by introducing the concept of "intersectional stigma" to examine the lives of sixteen women of color from Detroit, Michigan, who were drug users and HIV positive. And, in my own work (Dworkin 2005), I was the first to apply intersectional thinking to HIV/AIDS-prevention interventions and to ask why interventions were so focused on gender as a singular axis alone (without considerations of race, class, and sexualities). In the area of public health in 2005, Gentry, Elifson, and Sterk (2005) sought to use Hill-Collins's notion of intersectionality from *Black Feminist Thought* (Hill-Collins 1986, 1990) to aim for "more relevant" HIV/AIDS prevention among different groups of women at risk of HIV in Georgia, such as the "absolute homeless," "the rooming housed" (a step away from absolute homelessness), and the "hustling homeless." The work of Gentry, Elifson, and Sterk (2005) underscores that welfare-to-work and public housing were dismantled at the same time that the crack cocaine industry came to replace many low-wage jobs in high-risk environments and hence securing safe, affordable housing should be a goal of HIV/AIDS prevention for such groups. In 2006, the first book dedicated to intersectionality and health was written in the field of public health, an edited volume titled *Gender, Race, Class, and Health: Intersectional Approaches* (Schultz & Mullings 2006).

Early on, feminist thinkers were clear that intersectionality did not mean that we can "add together" marginalized statuses to come up with the concept of individuals who are "more marginalized" than others (Hill-Collins 1990). Rather, individuals could simultaneously occupy the position of oppressor and oppressed (Lorde 2007). And, some aspects of identity and structural experiences could be protective in a racist, sexist, classist, or homophobic world, while others would exacerbate harms.

Some work in public health, which exemplifies this latter principle, comes from Ilan Meyer's research (2003), conducted when he was at Columbia's Mailman School of Public Health. He was interested in the ways in which marginalized status—in his work, gay and lesbian identity—might be internalized to affect "minority stress." Simultaneously, however, he acknowledges that minority status can be a source of strength, for example, in the ways gays and lesbians find comfort from one another to diminish stigma or to form a strong sense of community that is a source of strength in a more hostile outside world. This is not unlike earlier findings within multiracial feminist studies of family, where feminist notions of an oppressive state of family relations have been challenged by women of color, who have argued that families work together to combat racism in external society (Thornton-Dill 1988). When intersectionality is applied to an understanding of how multiple social locations impact health, it has become increasingly clear that much more than "race" or "gender" or "class" or "sexuality" matter—some combination of all of these do.

Intersectionality and the HIV/AIDS Epidemic

Intersectionality is crucial to understanding the HIV epidemic and should be central to prevention interventions. I'll walk through this claim first for women and then for men. Not all women pay the costs of HIV equally in terms of "high-risk heterosexual contact" (the language used by the CDC). As I mentioned in chapter 1, it is Black and African American women who are paying far more with incident (new) HIV cases and death due to AIDS than White and Latina women. Overall, the HIV epidemic is remarkably racialized. While 13 percent of the female population in the United States is Black and/or African American, Black women constituted 65% of the HIV cases reported among women in

2013. In 2013, Latina women constituted 15% of the female population in the United States, and Latina women made up 17% of the reported cases among women, while White females constituted 65% of the female population in the United States and made up 17% of the HIV cases among women (CDC 2013c). In fact, African American women have the fourth highest rate of HIV infection in the United States, behind Black MSM, White MSM, and Latino/Hispanic MSM (2013a). In terms of deaths, while HIV is the ninth leading cause of death for White women ages twenty-five to forty-four, for African American women HIV is the third leading cause of death (CDC 2013d).

From the early days of the epidemic, the virus was definitely affecting the poorest and most marginalized women (Exner et al. 2003; Kamb & Wortley 2000). A racialized pattern has continued, with 34.8 new infections per 100,000 among Black women, 7.0 among Latino women, 9.3 among women who identify as having multiple races, 7.3 among Native Hawaiian/Other Pacific Islander, 5.1 among American Indian or Alaska Native, 2.2 among Asians, and 1.8 among White women (CDC 2013c). As one can see from this data, the rate of HIV among African American women is more than nineteen times the rate for White women and is approximately five times higher than for Latina women and Native Hawaiian/Other Pacific Islander women (CDC 2013c).

When one examines race and gender interactions, the results are also striking with respect to the need to recognize intersectionality. Of the men with HIV in the United States, 42% are Black, 30% are White, 23% are Hispanic, 2% are Asian, 2% are mixed race, less than 1% are Native Hawaiian or other Pacific Islander, and less than 1% are American Indian or Alaska Native (CDC 2013c). Of the women with HIV, 63% are Black, 17% are White, 17% are Hispanic, 2% are Asian, 2% are mixed race, 1% are American Indian or Alaska Native, and less than 1% are Native Hawaiian or other Pacific Islander (CDC 2013c). Thus race, class, gender, and sexuality intersect to produce a much larger category of risk for African American women concerning the total proportion of HIV cases compared to other women.

Why does this surveillance data matter for social scientists interested in inequality and health? Because if we think about science-based prevention interventions and think about the way that theory currently informs behavioral HIV-prevention interventions, we see that evidence-based programs often intervene with women at the individual level (or small-group level) and use a "gender norms" frame and not an intersectional one. Where race and gender are examined at once in the same evidence-based intervention (e.g., DiClemente et al. 2004; Wingood et al. 2004), then this is done through individual "race" or "gender" "pride" sessions, and there are no structural prevention interventions available in the Centers for Disease Control evidence-based interventions that wrestle with racism, poverty, homelessness, and gender inequality. The only "structural" evidence-based intervention listed on the CDC website is a condom distribution program (CDC 2013f).

Intersectionality involves not just race but also region of the country. African American women and men in the Northeast and Southeast are disproportionately affected by HIV (CDC 2012; Stratford et al. 2008). While the rate of new infections in the United States is highest in the northeastern United States, the U.S. South is home to 45–48% of the new infections in the United States, and southerners constitute 40% of the people living with HIV/AIDS (Kaiser Family Foundation 2012a, 2012b). Ten states account for two-thirds of HIV diagnoses, and seven of the top ten states by rate are in the southeastern United States (Kaiser Family Foundation 2012a). The District of Columbia (Washington, DC) has by far the highest rate of HIV, with 177.9 people per 100,000 infected in 2011—residents in the area identify HIV as the top problem in the area (Kaiser Family Foundation 2012b). The rate of HIV in D.C. is as high as it is in several developing nations.

Of persons who died from HIV infection from 1987 through 2009, the percentage who lived in the South increased from 28% to 54% while the percentage in the Northeast dropped from 39% to 22% and the percentage in the Midwest remained relatively stable, ranging from 8% to 11% (CDC 2011). Regional distributions of HIV also show us how important intersectionality is. This is the case because high rates of HIV in the southeastern part of the country are said to result from a combination of poverty, residential segregation, racism, gender inequality, STD rates, dense networks with a high HIV prevalence, men who have sex with men and women but who may not disclose their status to partners, women who have multiple partners, concurrency, and an uneven sex ratio of women to men given that numerous men circulate into and out of the prison system, where HIV rates are higher than in the general population (Adimora et al. 2003, 2004; Campbell 1995; Fullilove 2006). According to the Centers for Disease Control (CDC), a 2010 study that they carried out "concluded that there was no statistically significant difference in infection or prevalence by race or ethnicity among" the inner-city poor. "That is, people of color are disproportionately affected by HIV/AIDS because they are more likely to be poor and not because of their race/ethnicity" (Cawthorne 2010).

Age is also critical to recognition of why intersectionality matters for the HIV epidemic. Age also plays a key role in driving women's—and men's—HIV risks. While overall numbers of women and men with HIV are approximately equal, in young people ages thirteen to nineteen, a much greater proportion of HIV infections occurs among females (CDC 2002a, 2012). In South Africa (the focus of chapters 4 and 5), age intersects with gender profoundly: women in the 20–24-year age group have more than four times the HIV prevalence of males in the same age group—approximately 5.1% of young men in the 20–24-year age group are infected while 21.1% of young women are infected (Medical Research Council 2009; UNAIDS 2012). In the 25–29 age group, women have twice the HIV prevalence of males—32.7% of women are infected with HIV, 15.7% of men. At the same time, in the 35–39 age category, men have a greater proportion of HIV infections—24.8% of men and 18.5% of women are infected (Medical Research Council 2009). Thus, the epidemic clearly follows lines of age, race, and social class, and transmission and infection are bound to social and economic relations of inequality and more. We must ask ourselves, then, why our solutions to HIV so often lack a conceptualization of intersectional inequalities.

The intersection of race, class, gender, and sexuality is also brought to the fore when we examine new cases of HIV among Black men who have sex with men. From 2001 to 2006, cases among Black MSM rose 93% in thirty-three of fifty states in the United States (MMWR 2011). The HIV rates among Black MSM are astonishingly high—a study of 1,767 MSM in five U.S. cities carried out by the Centers for Disease Control found that 46% of Black MSM were infected (Voelker 2008). Another study carried out in seven urban centers in the United States found an HIV prevalence of 26% among young African American MSM compared to 7% among Latino MSM and 3% among White MSM (Bingham et al. 2003). Peterson and Jones (2009) now report that African

American MSM have not only the highest rates of HIV infection but also the highest rates of unknown infection—and their HIV incidence rates are on par with HIV rates in the general population in some developing countries.

The intersection between sexuality and race is critical to consider when thinking about the HIV epidemic and how to intervene through prevention interventions. Researchers have found consistently that Black MSM are less likely to identify as gay than White or other MSM and are more likely to engage in sex with both women and men than in other racial/ethnic groups (Miller et al. 2005; Dodge, Jeffries, & Sandfort 2008; Voelker 2008). In one study of gay-, bisexually, and heterosexually identified MSM, a significantly greater proportion of MSM who identified as heterosexual were African American than were White or Latino. In another study examining the concordance of sexual behavior and identity in a multiethnic sample of men and women, African American men had one of the highest proportions of discordance (that is, heterosexual identity and bisexual behavior) compared to other racial/ethnic groups represented in the study (Ross, Essien et al. 2003). In a meta-analysis of studies on African American MSM, research shows that Black MSM are more likely than White MSM to be bisexually active and less likely to disclose their same-sex activities to others (Millet et al. 2005). Additionally, in one study of five thousand African American gay-identified MSM, 22% of the men reported both male and female partners in the preceding five years (Montgomery et al. 2003). Unfortunately, "discrete categories of sexual identity used in targeted public health and HIV prevention campaigns (i.e., gay/homosexual, heterosexual, bisexual) may not adequately capture complexities underlying the sexuality of African-American men or groups of other men" (Ford et al. 2007, as cited in Saleh & Operario 2009, 390–91).

Assuming a discordance between identity and behavior means that we tend to adhere to the belief that there are three categories of sexuality and that men who have sex with men or with both women and men are "really gay" or "really bisexual" at the core (Saleh & Operario 2009). Many people therefore view the "discordance" between identity and behavior as being due to homophobia. Indeed, research finds that many Black men who have sex with men or with both women and men do not feel comfortable with a bisexual or a gay identity due to the enormous stigmas associated with these identities (Dodge, Jeffries, & Sandfort 2008). And, overall, rarely is bisexual identity even considered valid by many individuals in the United States, as it is often the case in U.S. society that constructions of sexuality borrow the "one-drop rule" and view any sexual activity between males as evidence of homosexuality, not bisexuality. Given the power of heteronormativity, combined with masculinity, religious influences, poverty, and disproportionate rates of incarceration where sex with men is not uncommon but may be taboo, it may not be surprising that it is very difficult for men to disclose anything other than a heterosexual identity.

However, even if we take the "discordance" between sexual identity and sexual behavior as "real," intersectionality is still helpful in aiding understanding of the risk and the prevention needs of such men. Research finds that this disjuncture may be due to the way racism and masculinity intersect to produce specific constructions of masculinity and sexuality that African American MSM adhere to. For example, research finds that African American men who have sex with men may not view their behavior as gay if they maintain the insertive or dominant role in penile-anal sex, feeling that this behavior is consistent with the sexual positioning of masculine heterosexual men (Fields, Fullilove, & Fullilove 2001; Fields et al. 2012; Malebranche et al. 2009). In addition, such men may view the receptive role as more feminine and therefore as more risky and may think that they are not at risk of HIV given that they may more often take the insertive role. Indeed, non-gay-identifying African American men who have sex with women and men are less likely to report receptive anal sex, according to some studies (Siegel et al. 2008).

Research also shows that African American MSM are influenced by broader ideals of masculinity in society, and given that they are already viewed as "less than a man" due to racism, they distance themselves from feminine gender expression more generally and may more frequently adhere to the idea that having multiple partners is masculine behavior (Fields et al. 2012; Malebranche et al. 2009). In new studies of young African American MSM, research finds that men prefer masculine partners, are uncomfortable with men who are more feminine playing an insertive role in sex, adhere to power dynamics wherein the more masculine partner makes condom-use decisions, and draw on perceived masculinity in partners in order to make risk determinations (Fields et al. 2012). Studies also show that racism in the gay community can contribute to African American men feeling greater disjuncture between their sexual feelings and their sexual identity; hence men may rely more on racialized masculinity than on sexuality as a way to maintain connection with African American communities (Saleh & Operario 2009; Teunis 2007).

Research also shows that Black MSM are more likely to partner with African American partners because racist social valuations, ideologies, and attitudes deem them to be less desirable partners, and thus their sexual networks are more narrow and dense and able to transmit HIV rapidly (their behavior may not be different than that of other MSM, but their networks have a higher seroprevalence—see Crosby et al. 2007; Millet et al. 2006, 2007; Harawa et al. 2004; Raymond & McFarlane 2009). They are also more likely to have age gaps in their partnerships than are members of other races, another factor in transmitting HIV/AIDS (Durant et al. 2007; Fields et al. 2012). And, partly due to class status and partly due to race disparities in health, they are less likely to be on antiretroviral therapy than White men, and hence, with higher viral loads, they may be more efficiently transmitting the virus (Millet et al. 2007). At the same time, several reviews have shown that they may be no more likely to engage in risky behavior than other MSM (Millett et al. 2007).

Public health scholars have been quite focused on comparing Black MSM to other racial groups in order to understand whether certain races have "risk factors" that explain their rates of HIV. For example, in his 2007 systematic review of the available literature, Millett found that Black MSM report less overall substance use than White MSM and have fewer sex partners and higher rates of STIs than White MSM (Millett et al. 2007). He found that their higher rates of HIV were not attributable to nongay identity, disclosure, or reported use of alcohol or drugs. In a new literature review, scholars now report that we can explain the differences in HIV rates between African American and White men through just a few variables—African American MSM are more likely to have an STI, are less likely to be on antiretroviral therapy, have less access to care and treatment services, and are more likely to be undiagnosed (Maulsby et al. 2013) (this set of findings sounds similar to the national AIDS policy focus).

Examining the data we have on the intersection of race and minority sexuality status matters for HIV risk not only among men who have sex with men (MSM) but also among men who have sex with both women and men (MSMW). Some research finds that there are important differences between Black MSMW and Black MSM: compared to Black MSM, Black MSMW do not identify as gay as often (are heterosexually identified more often), may not attend gay venues, and are more likely to be unemployed and have lower incomes than Black MSM (Spikes et al. 2009; Wheeler et al. 2008). Millet et al. (2005), in his review of MSM, described that African American heterosexually identified men report low rates of condom use, even among serodiscordant partners, more sexual partners, more involvement in concurrent partnerships, and a greater likelihood of having an STI than men in other racial or ethnic groups who are heterosexually identified.

Other research has suggested that non-gay-identifying African American MSMW who have sex with gay-identifying MSM are less likely to disclose a positive HIV serostatus to sexual partners before having unprotected sex than gay-identifying MSM (Millet et al. 2005; Mutchler et al. 2008), although other research vigorously challenges this frame as not only sensationalistic (i.e. "the down low" that implies "secret sex") but also inaccurate in terms of the highly variable and contextual disclosure behaviors that men enact (Mackenzie 2013; Malebranche et al. 2010; Saleh & Operario 2009; Sandfort & Dodge 2008). Indeed, researchers are thoroughly challenging notions of the "down low" by suggesting that such notions are consistent with a long history of racism, objectification, and suspicion placed on Black bodies, whereby both women and men are assumed to be sexually promiscuous and to have a dangerous sexuality in need of control (Hill-Collins 1990). Several researchers challenge notions of "secrecy" among Black MSM and MSMW, arguing that men (and women) of all racial and ethnic groups hold "secrets" and because research focuses so frequently on how Black men are "different" from other men, researchers are continuing to exoticize and marginalize men of color in the HIV epidemic.

Intersectionality as a concept helps us to understand how "coming out" as gay or bisexual may not be possible for Black MSMW, nor may it be desirable, nor is it even viewed as an accurate indicator of sexual identity, although homophobia may still play a role in self-identification among some men (Mackenzie 2013). Several other reasons for less gay identification among African American MSM compared to non–African American MSM have been articulated, including a fear of stigma and/or violence from homophobic African American communities (and beyond); gender norms; internalized conflict over religious/moral beliefs and same-sex desire; internalized homophobia; a masculinized performance of Black manhood for self-protection and because it is one of a few resources to draw upon; desire for children; and disproportionate incarceration rates and situational MSM behavior (Malebranche 2008; Malebranche et al. 2009; Millett et al. 2005, 2007).

The reason all of this data is so critical to understand is this: it is not simply the case, as has already been mentioned, that men who are heterosexually identified within the HIV/AIDS epidemic have been viewed by researchers as perpetrators of oppression of women in a gender order, but it is also the case that bisexually identified or bisexually behaving men are also experiencing race, class, and sexuality marginalizations—or disjunctures between sexual acts and sexual identities—that shape their HIV risks. However, instead of being viewed as vulnerable to HIV, they are often viewed as the responsible "bridges" through which more innocent women or other men are made "vulnerable" (Kalichman et al. 1998; Kahn et al. 1997; Malebranche et al. 2010; Millett et al. 2005; Sandfort & Dodge 2008; Stokes et al. 1996). This is unfortunate, as new research (Dodge et al. 2012; Malebranche et al. 2009; Malebranche et al. 2010) reveals that men who have sex with both women and men enact variable sexual behaviors and identities (and their intersection is variable as well), and have highly variable condom use depending on perceptions of risk (based on partner type, whether casual or long-term and whether male or female). Men who have sex with women and men also have highly variable disclosure behaviors depending on a large number of factors that are partly but not yet fully understood.

Finally, heterosexually active men who identify as heterosexual and do not have sex with men are also impacted by the intersection of race, class, gender, and sexuality when it comes to HIV risk. In chapter 1, I pointed out that "heterosexually identified men" tend to structure sex according to a hydraulic model of male desire, the predominance of penile-vaginal penetration, the centrality of male pleasure, and an understanding of masculinity as bolstered by multiple partners (Exner et al. 2003; Flood 2003a, 2003b; Holland et al. 1994a, 1994b; Kimmel 1995; Vittelone 2000). Relatively recent qualitative focus-group research with heterosexually identified African American men in the United States shows that such men are influenced by two specific masculine ideologies—that Black men should have sex with multiple women and that men should not be gay or bisexual (Bowleg et al. 2011). In addition, this research project showed that men did not feel able to refuse sexual opportunities because these opportunities helped men to self-constitute as masculine, and this was the case even if the sex was known to be risky (Bowleg et al. 2011).

Thus, within existing HIV-prevention interventions, sexuality and race are perhaps treated all too often as identity-based categories that intersect to produce HIV risks or "problematic" choices, but it is also critical to think about how structures of inequality shape men's HIV risks. Domestically, as we underscored in Higgins, Hoffman, and Dworkin 2010, a host of contextual and structural factors amalgamate to heighten heterosexually active men's risk of HIV, including residential segregation, unstable housing and homelessness, unemployment, migratory work, and high rates of incarceration among men of color (Adimora, Schoenbach, & Floris-Moore 2009; Fullilove 2006). Ninety-three percent of prisoners in the United States are men, and African American men are seven times as likely to be incarcerated as White men (Golembeski & Fullilove 2005; USDOJ 2006). Among the incarcerated, the AIDS rate is up to four or five times higher than in the general population.

As sociologists know, massive shifts towards deindustrialization have economically destabilized millions of inner-city men of color, dramatically increasing the size of the urban underclass and, due to a lack of options for work and harsh "three strikes" drug laws, the prison population (Wilson 1987, 1996). These demographic shifts contribute to more labor migration or circular migration through the prison system (Fullilove 2006). Yet in interventions on HIV risk, it is a gender frame that is privileged for women while HIV-prevention interventions in the funded science base (NIH/CDC) have not often intervened to change the context of deindustrialization, joblessness, residential segregation, and the prison industrial complex—all of which increase men's vulnerability to HIV (for one exception of a "structurally informed" intervention in the

United States, see Raj et al. 2013). Nor has HIV-prevention-intervention work adequately examined the ways in which gender, race, and class inequalities have substantially shaped masculinity and HIV risks of men of color in the United States. If prevention work moves forward with only a "gender-specific" framework, we will continue to inadvertently view men as "causing" women's HIV/AIDS risks, and these men will disproportionately be racial/ethnic minority men or men of marginalized sexualities, who face resounding doses of race and class oppression (and for men who are not heterosexual, sexuality oppression) as part of their risks. Rather than frame these men as failed individual men who cannot treat women well enough or make essentializing assumptions that certain men cannot control their own desires for multiple sexual partners, we need to consider the ways in which structural inequalities interact with race, class, sexuality relations, and masculinities to arrive at solutions in HIV prevention.

In the United States, do any of the evidence-based HIV/AIDS-prevention interventions that I previously examined in chapter 1 take structural aspects of race and class inequalities and their attendant dynamics into account? No. Some studies that can be considered structural have been carried out with women, but not with men. There have been very few interventions that examine the intersection of poverty and HIV/AIDS in the United States, and those that do have not yet made it into the Centers for Disease Control Diffusion of Effective Behavioral Interventions (DEBI) program. There is only new study (Raj et al. 2013) that has been funded by the National Institutes of Health that is structurally informed and focused on housing, employment, and HIV risks—the results are promising but do not yet involve randomized trial results.

Does the available data that exists now tell us that structurally shifting women or men from a state of homelessness to more stable housing will offer some reduction in HIV/AIDS risks? The data certainly does suggest this—Angela Aidala and her colleagues (2005) found just that in their analysis of 2,149 clients at sixteen medical and social service sites. They found that the odds of recent drug use, needle use, or sex exchange at baseline was 204 times higher among the homeless and unstably housed than among persons with stable housing. And they show that changing housing status over time to an improved state of housing (from homeless to unstably housed or from unstably housed to stably housed) was significantly associated with reduced risk of drug use, needle use, needle sharing, and unprotected sex (a 50% reduction in these risks over and above those whose housing status did not improve). Elise Riley and colleagues (2007) make the same argument in their work in the Tenderloin district near the University of California–San Francisco and argue that calls for safer sex do not take constraining structures into account.

Furthermore, Kathy Sikkema and colleagues (2000) carried out a community-based intervention conducted in eighteen low-income inner-city developments in the United States. Housing developments were matched on the basis of demographic characteristics of tenants, and one of each pair was randomly assigned to the intervention condition. Women were encouraged to develop Health Councils to recruit other women into workshop series on reducing risks. At one-year follow-up, there was a significant reduction of unprotected intercourse in intervention communities compared to comparison housing projects. Consideration of intersectionality of many kinds (age, race, sexuality, region) should be structured into HIV prevention interventions in the United States and worldwide. While the epidemiological information that I covered in this chapter reveals the clear importance of an intersectional framework, evidence-based prevention interventions tend to be structured around "gender norms" or "racial pride" or "sexuality." Intersectionality focused on both identity and structures will be crucial to tailoring prevention interventions around the needs of target populations in the future, and we will look back at our reliance on single risk categories with surprise at the simplicity of our methods.

A final problematic issue that impacts HIV prevention interventions in the United States is that our current surveillance categories are singular and hierarchical and encourage us to privilege singular "risks." To be specific, within the United States, there is a reliance on *singular risk categories* (e.g., heterosexual, MSM, IDU—all are behaviorally defined) and this is coupled with *hierarchical risk assessment* (of the risks that a person presents with, the "highest" risk behavior determines his or her classification). Under this classification system, anal sex has the highest risk, penile-vaginal sex is next, injection drug use is next, oral sex is next, and sex between two women is viewed as having the lowest probability of transmission. A woman who has sex with women and men, and whose female partner is an IDU, will be categorized as having heterosexual-transmission risks. One could be a woman who has always had long sessions of oral sex with multiple HIV-positive women but who has had one episode of heterosexual contact, and one would be counted as having heterosexual risk. A bisexual female who does not use drugs and has sex with a man will be counted as having a heterosexual-transmission risk.

This classification system can erroneously conflate sexual act with sexual identity. A gay man can have sex with a gay woman, and this would be counted as a heterosexual sex risk. A bisexual woman who has anal sex with a gay man will be classified as having heterosexual-transmission risks. A woman who has sex with women and men where the male partner is an IDU will be classified as having sex with an intravenous drug user, and this will be placed into a "heterosexual-transmission" category (CDC 2013e). Thus, one can see that "heterosexual sex" is used quite often as a risk category even if the sex is "gay" or "queer" because sexual acts and not identities matter in the CDC risk-classification system. While focused on behaviors and avoiding the messy problems of identity, this reliance can miss the "risks" of bisexually identified women and men, transgender women and men, and several other groups that may experience disjunctures between their sexual acts and their sexual identities.

Surveillance categories do not often get reported at the intersection of several identities or behaviors and therefore do not facilitate easy analysis of the contextual factors that shape risk aside from "heterosexual transmission," "IDU," or "MSM" (Young & Meyer 2005). The resultant effect of singular, hierarchical categories is clear in prevention-intervention research and is linked to my arguments in this chapter about a lack of intersectionality in HIV-prevention interventions. That is, much HIV-prevention work on heterosexually active women is "gender specific" and is structured by early social science assumptions of a gender order wherein women are viewed as oppressed and men are considered powerful perpetrators who benefit in the gender order and cause women's HIV. Indeed, some HIV researchers have cautioned against the privileging of any one aspect of identity or behavior or of a unified community or contextual "aspect" of practice as being the "key" organizing principle for HIV-prevention interventions, given that such an assumption may be seriously flawed (Bowleg 2012; Watkins-Hayes 2014).

At the same time, it is often men of color who are viewed as the "responsible" bridges for women's HIV risk. As Millett and colleagues adeptly pointed out (2005),

> there needs to be clarification around whether the primary source of HIV infection among black women is black men who are bisexually active or black men who are heterosexually active. The best population based estimates of black MSM show that only 3% of all black men ages 18–49 were homosexually or bisexually-active. In contrast, a population estimate of high risk black heterosexuals found that 29.7% of exclusively heterosexual black men ages 18–49 engages in high-risk sexual activities. Assuming that 97% of all black men in the United States are exclusively heterosexual and that 30% of these men engage in high risk activity, a central issue emerges: Are heterosexually transmitted cases of HIV in black women driven by a small percentage of MSMW who have a high prevalence of HIV and unknown HIV risk behavior, or by a much larger population of exclusively heterosexual black men who have comparatively lower HIV prevalence but high HIV risk behavior? (57)

The research base does not yet make the answer to this question clear, but it does point to the dangers of privileging a singular understanding of the linkages within the sex-gender-sexuality triad.

The limitations that come with privileging this singular understanding of the sex-gender-sexuality triad was discussed in Higgins, Hoffman, and Dworkin (2010), where we argued that

> [d]espite its focus on how gender socialization and gendered structures shape women's susceptibility to HIV, the vulnerability paradigm fails to address how masculinity and the intersection of various structural forces (e.g., class, race, and global inequalities) shape heterosexually active men's HIV risk. The paradigm has also perpetuated unfortunate gendered tropes, such as sexual protectionism of women, a discounting of women's pleasure and agency, and the belief that women are motivated to prevent HIV through condoms but men are not and (with a few exceptions) that men have multiple partners but women do not. Heterosexual men are disadvantaged by a model that negates men's health risks and fails to address how masculinity can be harmful to their own—and women's—health. (441)

Intersectional frameworks may not provide a total solution, but this conceptual turn could begin to bring some populations, behaviors, and identities into clearer view while allowing for much-needed contextual understandings of "at risk" and "vulnerable" and prevention solutions.

Historical and contemporary research has already shown that responses to disease do not simply reflect the reality of a disease but also constitute it (Patton 1990, 2002; Treichler 1988, 1999a, 1999b). We must therefore continually be self-reflexive as to how HIV-prevention efforts might be uncritically bolstering limited linkages in a sex-gender-sexuality triad that lead to (1) failure to perceive heterosexually active men's vulnerability to sexual risks; (2) lack of attention to the ways in which race, class, gender and sexuality intersect among the men who are most affected by HIV; (3) lumping of MSM and MSMW into one category (MSM) because inconsistencies between self-identity and behavior are glossed over and differential condom-use practices with male and female partners (or short-term and long-term partners) are erased; and (4) overdetermined visibility of heterosexually active women as vulnerable and as subject to HIV risk in a monolithic gender order wherein men are viewed as harming women and "causing" HIV (while data shows that in several epidemics, women having concurrent partners is common). It is time to nuance the gender order in HIV prevention and consider intersectionality in theory and in practice in prevention programming. Examining the simultaneity of race, class, and shifting gender relations for heterosexually active (and non–heterosexually active) women and men remains utterly vital, as does the ability to consider structural interventions for HIV prevention. In the next chapter, I will take the assumptions of the sex-gender-sexuality triad that are often deployed in HIV prevention and critically assess global health programs that intervene with women and men to reduce HIV and violence risks. I ask, why are there two separate tracks of work—one for heterosexually active women and one for heterosexually active men? What are the points of overlap, tension, synergy, and contradiction across these two lines of work? How can each be bolstered by drawing on the strengths of the other?

3

Women's Empowerment and Work with Men in HIV and Antiviolence Programs

Globally, approximately thirty-three million people are living with HIV/ AIDS, and nearly 50% of infected people worldwide are now women, up from 35% in 1985 (UNAIDS 2008, 2012). In most, but not all, regions of the world, women and girls represent an increasing proportion of people living with HIV/AIDS, and that proportion is expected to increase, especially in sub-Saharan Africa, Asia, Russia, and Latin America (UNAIDS 2012). Additionally, UNAIDS reports detail that in several countries, 50% of new infections were transmitted between spouses (UNAIDS 2012). Finally, research is clear that the epidemics of HIV and violence are synergistic—each exacerbating the effects of the other and each undergirded by relations of gender inequality.

Research frequently points to the need to empower women in order to effectively combat the twin epidemics of HIV/AIDS and gender-based violence. Simultaneously, unlike with the domestic U.S. epidemic, there has been increased global attention to working with heterosexually active men in gender-equality efforts—these approaches intervene in constructions of masculinities as part of the fight against HIV/AIDS and violence. No research except for my own has considered these two lines of research side by side to assess the promises and limitations of these separate tracks of work (Dworkin et al. 2011). And no research has considered how there are points of overlap, synergies, tensions, and contradictions between these two approaches. In this chapter, I analyze these two parallel lines of work by examining a gendered power/ women's empowerment strategy that seeks to reduce women's violence and HIV risks by integrating economic empowerment and HIV prevention through the use of microfinance programming. I then examine the promise of gender-transformative programs with men (those that seek to challenge men to reflect on the "costs of masculinity" to men and women—and to transform masculinities to be more gender equitable) for reducing violence and HIV risks. I ask, what are the promises, limitations, and unintended consequences of each line of work? How can researchers and practitioners capitalize on the synergies that come from bolstering each line of work with the strengths of the other?

As I argued in chapters 1 and 2, research is clear that sexual- and reproductive-health outcomes, including violence and HIV risks, are shaped by broader gender inequalities within numerous realms, including the economic, social, interpersonal, cultural, and educational arenas (Dunkle et al. 2006; Dworkin & Ehrhardt 2007; Global Coalition on Women & AIDS 2006; Greig et al. 2008; Gupta 2002; Krishnan et al. 2008, 2010; Jewkes et al. 2010). Thus, a new generation of health programming is linking women's empowerment and health to reduce HIV and violence risk (Kim et al. 2007; Pronyk et al. 2005, 2006, 2008). Simultaneously, there is increased recognition that masculinities (socially constructed, institutionally supported, and collectively practiced sets of ideals that define what it means to be a man) can shape both women's and men's health (Courtenay 2000a, 2000b; Dworkin et al. 2012; Flood et al. 2010; Jewkes & Morrell 2010; Morrell et al. 2013; Sabo & Gordon 1995). Recent global health interventions have therefore attempted to reshape the norms and practices of masculinities that contribute to HIV/ AIDS and gender-based violence (Barker, Ricardo, & Nascimento 2007; Dunkle & Jewkes 2007; Flood et al. 2010; Kalichman et al. 2007, 2008; Population Council 2006; Sonke Gender Justice Network 2007).

What has been so fascinating to me over the course of my career is the fact that these are two distinct (and separate) approaches within HIV and antiviolence programming—one is centered on women's empowerment and is specifically focused on working with women, and one seeks to work with men for gender equality in the name of improved health outcomes. In a 2011 article that I published in the *American Journal of Public Health* with my colleagues Megan Dunbar, Suneeta Krishnan, Abbey Hatcher, and Sharif Sawires, I noted that both approaches have much in common. For example, both tracks of work acknowledge that gender inequalities are drivers of the HIV and violence epidemics. Both tracks of work therefore tend to take a "gender-transformative" approach that attempts to change gender norms and roles and promote more equitable relationships between women and men. However, there are differences between the two approaches, and there are some hidden assumptions within these two lines of work that should be elucidated in order for the field to wrestle with key questions as these lines of work progress forward. Namely, what are the strengths and limitations of these programs that are on separate tracks—one pitched to women and one largely targeting men? To what extent does one line of work enhance or inhibit the goals of the other? How can the weaknesses of these approaches be minimized and the synergies between the two approaches be leveraged such that gains in HIV/AIDS and antiviolence programs can be achieved?

In order to understand the promises and limitations of each of these tracks of work, it is quite critical to briefly review what may be obvious to the reader—that women's empowerment programs work with women and leave men out of the intervention. Women's empowerment programming borrows from the logic of the sex-gender-sexuality triad that has been examined in previous chapters, treating biological women as being subject to gender inequality in a sex-gender system that is linked to heterosexuality. Here, it is thought that since women are disempowered through gender inequality more broadly and gender relations in marriage or other partnerships, they need to be empowered. To become more empowered, this line of work discusses that women need more education, economic power, sexuality education, sexual and reproductive rights, cultural visibility, decision-making control, household bargaining power, violence prevention, and safer-sex negotiating power. Female-initiated methods such as female condoms and microbicides (gels to prevent HIV that are placed inside the vagina or anus) were in fact developed, in part, because male condoms are viewed as being in the direct control of men (Stein 1990). The literature suggests that women need greater agency to protect themselves from HIV and greater control over resources such as income, land, property, health services, food security, education, and housing that can shape relationship power and thus safer sex negotiations (Action AIDS International 2006; Dworkin et al. 2013; Gollub 2000; Gupta 2001, 2002; Weiser et al. 2007).

Work with men to improve gender equality and health has also generally been a single-sex line of work and has generally, though not always, left women out of its programming. These programs have tended to take two main approaches and have either (a) sought to "partner with men" to improve women's health outcomes or (b) sought to "transform gender relations" to be less inequitable by focusing on shifting the norms and practices of masculinity that contribute to negative health outcomes and gender inequality. Overall, in this approach, men are encouraged to rethink gender-related beliefs and practices and are engaged to help resolve gender inequalities and work towards the empowerment of women to achieve improvements in health. Men have been addressed in this way not only in science-based prevention interventions but also through numerous international conferences, United Nations meetings, global networks, and white papers that seek to reduce violence and HIV risks among women and men (Wegner et al. 1997; Barker, Ricardo, & Nascimento 2007; Flood 2003b; Greig 2003; Hutchinson et al. 2004; International AIDS Alliance 2003; Peacock 2002; Peacock et al. 2009; Pile et al. 1999; Pulerwitz, Martin, et al. 2010; Rivers & Aggleton 1999; Stern, Peacock, & Alexander 2009; UNAIDS 2000, 2001).

In order to flesh out the first approach, which is the women's empowerment approach, I will first lay out background information that will help readers to more deeply understand some basics about programs and their promises and limitations. First, it is critical to remind that most HIV-prevention interventions in the science base (another reminder: when I state "science-base," I mean those funded research programs that are supported by the National Institutes of Health and the Centers for Disease Control) tend to focus on individuals and small groups, although some emphasis has also been placed at the community level. As I noted in the last chapter, there have been fewer interventions that have been developed as "structural interventions"—those that reshape the contexts in which risk is enacted. Examples of structural interventions not only include economic empowerment, livelihood (agriculture and food security), housing, and property-rights interventions but also include community mobilization, the integration of HIV-prevention and family-planning services, contingent funding interventions (paying families or households on the basis of performing a certain health behavior, such as making a preventive doctor appointment), and educational interventions that keep girls in school (Auerbach & Adimora 2010; Blankenship, Bray, & Merson 2000; Blankenship et al. 2006; Gupta et al. 2008; Parker, Easton, & Klein 2000). These approaches are thought to provide more enduring protection than individual and small-group interventions because these programs change the nature of the environment to reshape contexts of risk, facilitating different behavioral choices.

Before we focus on the integration of HIV prevention and women's economic empowerment through microfinance and microenterprise, it is important to highlight that microfinance and the microenterprise development industries have had a long history both in the United States and worldwide. There have been several sociological books written about the development of these industries both in the United States (Jurik 2005) and globally (Karim 2011; Roy 2010; Sanyal 2014). These texts not only underscore the ideologies within the microenterprise industry and shape its internal practices (e.g., Jurik 2005 is focused on the emergence of the industry in the United States in the context of welfare-to-work policies and the way programs changed over time in light of pressures to be fiscally self-sustaining and profitable) but also underscore its massive level of variability. Karim and Roy focus on microfinance for its linkages to globalization, structural adjustment, the global financial crisis, gender relations, and power relations between the global North and the global South. These analyses are incisive, although their critiques of microfinance and microenterprise development have not yet made their way into HIV/AIDS prevention studies much yet (for exceptions, see Dworkin & Blankenship 2009).

In order to provide readers with some background information on how the field of HIV prevention came to embrace microfinance and microenterprise, it is critical to offer some history on the income-generation industry itself. Muhammad Yunus is often credited publicly with the development and implementation of the concepts of microfinance and microcredit. He is an economist and is the founder of Grameen Bank, which attempts to create social and economic development for the poor "from below." His work has been publicly credited with substantially reducing poverty in Bangladesh. He obtained a Ph.D. in economics, taught in the United States, and then returned to Bangladesh in 1972 to find that most of the population was facing famine and was in poverty. He wanted to find out what caused poverty, and taking a rather innovative methodological tactic for a Ph.D. in economics, he walked into villages and asked villagers face-to-face questions about their situation. He listened to villagers' voices and responses and concluded that a lack of access to credit is what kept many in poverty.

Yunus therefore came up with the idea of microcredit in 1972 when he loaned forty-two women who were bamboo stool makers twenty-seven dollars from his own pocket, only to be paid back with interest, giving birth to the microfinance industry. Since its formation, Grameen has experienced enormous growth and now serves 8.4 million members, more than 95% of whom are women (Bornstein 2013). In his book *Banker to the Poor,* he states that societies can achieve "gender equality through the empowerment of women" (Yunus 2003) and focuses on the mechanism of poverty reduction to meet that aim. Indeed, microfinance (MF) programs represent a range of programs that seek to alleviate poverty by providing access to credit, savings, or business skills. Such programs, which usually involve small amounts of money, are especially vital for the poor, particularly women in poverty, who are often excluded from educational opportunities, highly valued job skills, and traditional financial institutions and services (Jurik 2005; Pearson 2001; Sanyal 2014).

It is important to keep in mind that microfinance programs are highly varied, but

> some frequent features include group lending (small groups are formed voluntarily, loans are made to individuals within the groups, but all members are held responsible for loan repayment); progressive lending and dynamic incentives (loan size is increased with successful loan repayment); frequent and almost immediate loan repayment schedule; (often) compulsory savings (a portion of the loan placed in a group fund and strict rules for withdrawal applied); and either no collateral required or collateral substitutes permitted. (Dworkin & Blankenship 2009, 462)

Indeed, such programs are not static and have changed with time. MF institutions later added to the above basic program structures and services by providing more flexible loan repayment, a variety of savings options, business development services, and, in some instances, pension plans and insurance (debt relief with death of borrower, health insurance, natural disaster insurance) (Sengupta & Aubuchon 2008; Sievers & Vandenberg 2007).

It is interesting to point out that empowerment discourse for women is strongly linked to microfinance, microcredit, and microenterprise development and emerged long before HIV/AIDS researchers and practitioners became interested in it. According to Mayoux (2005),

> The problem of women's access to credit was given particular emphasis at the first International Women's Conference in Mexico in 1975 as part of the emerging awareness of the importance of women's productive role both for national economies, and for women's rights. This led to the setting up of the Women's World Banking network and production of manuals for women's credit provision. Other women's organizations world-wide set up credit and savings components both as a way of increasing women's incomes and bringing women together to address wider gender issues. From the mid-1980s there was a mushrooming of donor, government and NGO-sponsored credit programmes in the wake of the 1985 Nairobi women's conference. Support for targeting women in microfinance programmes comes from organizations of widely differing political perspectives. There has recently been an apparent convergence of policy and terminology and common concerns with sustainability, participation and empowerment as donor agencies and NGOs have attempted to address their critics, and activists have become engaged in constructive dialogue. (3)

Discourses of empowerment as linked to microfinance were further reinforced by the 1997 MicroCredit Summit in Washington, DC, which listed "reaching and empowering women" as a second goal after poverty reduction. A large expansion in targeting women as clients in microfinance ensued because women are disproportionately in poverty and they have excellent repayment rates relative to men. These programs were thought to lead not only to the economic empowerment of women but also to their social empowerment. With increased income, it was thought that women's well-being would improve and that with increased well-being for both women and their families, programs were assumed to "initiate a series of virtuous spirals" that include "wider social and political empowerment" (Mayoux 2005). The year 2005 was deemed the "year of microcredit," and microfinance for women is now seen as a key strategy in meeting not only Millennium Goal 1—eradicating extreme poverty—but also Millennium Development Goal 3—promoting gender equality and empowering women.

While antipoverty goals were sought as a form of women's empower-ment early on in the development of microenterprise and microfinance, other global disciplines and realms soon became interested in this devel-opment, wondering if the empowering gains that were associated with poverty-reduction efforts could yield health benefits. For example, in the 1990s and 2000s, advocates and researchers in reproductive health, family planning, and child nutrition, as well as antiviolence advocates, sought to understand whether women's participation in microfinance programs improved outcomes in a variety of areas, including contracep-tive use, violence against women, health bargaining power, public status, and mobility.

While there are various methodological shortcomings of microfi-nance (MF) and microenterprise studies (Dworkin & Hatcher 2012), several studies to date have found that MF participation leads to in-creased reproductive-health decision-making power (contraceptive use for fertility decisions and family planning). Schuler & Hashemi (1994) found the same in a study of MF participants in rural Bangladesh. Simi-larly, qualitative work by Hays-Mitchell (1999) in Peru also found that women report having more control over fertility decisions (timing/spac-ing of births of children) after participating in a credit program. These authors all suggest that some women find that a source of income gives them a platform of increased power from which to negotiate with male partners. These and other studies in the health field signaled to HIV/AIDS researchers that it may be wise to assess whether programs that sought to minimize women's economic dependencies on men and em-power them economically may positively impact their HIV risks.

Poverty reduction plays a central role in women's empowerment discourse within the HIV/AIDS-prevention realm. Numerous domes-tic events have been held over the last nine years that highlight a trend of increasing research interest at the intersection of microfinance and HIV prevention. Domestically, in March of 2006, the CDC held a con-sultation on microfinance that centered on the southeastern United States. Out of this consultation, a paper was published that called for the need to examine microfinance/microenterprise (ME) as an HIV-risk-reduction strategy (Stratford et al. 2008). The HIV portion of the CDC has yet to put out a call for proposals for researchers to develop, imple-ment, and test such an intervention.

In July of 2007, Yale University's Center for Interdisciplinary Research on AIDS hosted a similar workshop that emphasized both domestic and international settings and examined whether microfinance influenced other health outcomes beyond HIV/AIDS. The workshop was titled "Microfinance and Beyond: Structural Interventions Promoting Economic Opportunity as HIV Risk Reduction." Several published papers emerged out of this workshop as well (Dworkin & Blankenship 2009; Hanck, West, & Tsui 2007; Smoyer & Patterson 2007). Additionally, the numerous international AIDS conferences showcase new research projects that examine how microfinance assists HIV-infected households, reduces stigma against those with HIV/AIDS, and empowers women to protect themselves. Of course, microfinance received even more public acclaim in 2006 when Muhammad Yunus won the Nobel Peace Prize for his work with Grameen Bank in Bangladesh. And, in 2011–2012, the Centers for Disease Control partnered with CommonHealth Action and the San Francisco State Institute for Health Equity to develop a sustainable and adaptable microenterprise intervention in the United States to address social and economic determinants of HIV/AIDS, STDs, and sexual violence. There is much interest in this topic, clearly.

At first glance, it may seem to readers that an emphasis on economic empowerment as an HIV-prevention strategy is urgent. Research findings indicate that economically disempowered women and girls who are dependent on male partners financially are more likely to be constrained into sexually risky situations: less able to negotiate safer sex with partners, less likely to be able to leave an abusive or violent relationship (which also increases HIV risks), and much more likely to exchange sex for material goods, food, shelter, or assets (Dworkin & Blankenship 2009; Dworkin et al. 2013; Exner et al. 2003; Gupta & Weiss 1993; Hallman 2004; Tsai, Hung, & Weiser 2012; Weiser et al. 2007). Research also shows that poverty affects girls and women more negatively than boys and men with regard to unsafe sex and that economic independence for women is an important predictor of their being able to negotiate safer sex (Grieg & Koopman 2003; Hallman 2004). In short, situations of risk are fostered within contexts of economic disadvantage and dependency, particularly when coupled with laws, cultural practices, and sexual norms that disempower women relative to men (Grabe 2010, 2012; Hallman 2004; Lu et al. 2013).

While the mechanisms through which microfinance may work to reduce women's HIV risks are not well explored, a few key mechanisms
have been hypothesized. First, improvements in women's income are
thought to reshape women's household decision-making power. This is
believed to increase women's clout and bargaining power, which can help
them to negotiate safer sex or reshape their household status such that
their experiences of violence decrease. Second, improvements in women's
income help them to secure goods, food, shelter, or other needs-based
materials, and if their asset base increases, they are less likely to turn to
the exchange of sex for these items in situations of dire poverty, food insecurity, and disinheritance, or in other constrained circumstances. Third,
increased income and the skills that are taught in income-generation programs may improve women's self-confidence, self-efficacy, or other psychosocial outcomes that may act as mediators or moderators to reduce
their HIV risks. And, since economic dependencies between women and
men have been shown to foster gender inequality and, in some instances,
violence, improving women's economic position relative to men or the
economic position of the household is thought to potentially reduce
women's experiences of violence. As has already been noted in this book,
women who experience higher rates of violence are at greater risk of HIV
than women who do not experience violence.

Thus, even though (1) there is a recognized need for innovative structural interventions that help to prevent HIV/AIDS and violence; (2)
there is evidence for the relationship between gender inequality and the
spread of HIV/AIDS (and this has led to an increase in gender-specific
and gender-transformative HIV/AIDS-prevention interventions, several
of which were successful; see chapter 1); and (3) economic empowerment has repeatedly been named as a contextual factor that assists in
the prevention and mitigation of the disease, particularly for women
(Dworkin & Blankenship 2009; Kim et al. 2002; Kim & Watts 2005;
Manopaiboon et al. 2003; Zierler & Krieger 1997), shockingly little has
been done to promote the development of structural interventions that
integrate women's economic empowerment into HIV/AIDS-prevention
efforts (Dworkin & Blankenship 2009; Sherman et al. 2006; Stratford
et al. 2008). Domestically, this is particularly the case despite the fact
that, as I have already described, African American and Latina women
are disproportionately affected by HIV and the CDC has determined in

a 2010 study that poor people living in cities with a high HIV-infection rate were twice as likely to be infected as people with incomes above the poverty line in the same neighborhoods (Cawthorne 2010). Only two randomized controlled trials exist that test integrated HIV-prevention and economic-empowerment programs, and both are in developing countries (their results will be examined later in this chapter).

Now let's look at programs. One domestic pilot study (not a randomized trial) known as the JEWEL program (Jewelry Education for Women Empowering Their Lives) examined the efficacy of an integrated HIV/economic program for drug-using sex workers in Baltimore, Maryland (Sherman et al. 2006). The program offered six two-hour HIV-prevention sessions and assisted women with the making, marketing, and selling of jewelry. Using a pre-/post-test design, researchers found significant reductions both in the exchange of drugs or sex for money and in the median number of sex-trade partners per month. And, at three-month follow-up, income earned from the sale of jewelry was associated with a reduction in number of sex partners. Unfortunately, there was no control group in this study, and with a pre-/post-test design, it is difficult to ascertain whether it was the program content that changed individuals or whether particular individuals who were already more likely to change to begin with self-selected into the program and drove the positive results. Still, the fact that women's increased income drove a reduction in the number of sex partners shows that economic empowerment is a promising strategy to reduce HIV risks for some women.

Of the other programs that integrate HIV prevention and women's economic empowerment, only two randomized controlled trials have been conducted. The IMAGE Program (Intervention for Microfinance and Gender Equity) tested the effect of a curriculum that combined gender-equity, violence-prevention, and an HIV-prevention intervention with group-based microfinance. Based in rural Limpopo, South Africa, where it is known that there are high rates of HIV, high rates of violence against women, high levels of unemployment, and high levels of gender inequality, the program involved collaboration between the Small Enterprise Foundation (SEF), the Rural Aids and Development Action Research (RADAR) program, and the London School of Tropical Hygiene.

After ten sessions of a participatory curriculum called "Sisters for Life" in IMAGE, a smaller group of women received additional training to mobilize their community on issues related to intimate partner violence and HIV infection. This randomized controlled trial shows that IMAGE shifted multiple dimensions of women's empowerment (Kim et al. 2007) and increased participant use of voluntary counseling and testing for HIV (Pronyk et al. 2008). The effect of IMAGE on women's empowerment was significant when the program was later compared with groups receiving microfinance only (Kim et al. 2009), suggesting that microfinance has a synergistic effect when implemented alongside gender-equity content (and that it is less powerful without the gender-equity content).

Notably, the IMAGE program resulted in a 55% greater reduction in intimate partner violence at two-year follow-up for program participants than for the control group (Pronyk et al. 2006). What is less clear in the IMAGE example is how an intervention to empower women economically and in terms of gender equity shifted the incidence of violence by male partners who did not directly participate in the intervention. Several factors may have influenced the reported decline in violence, although the causal pathways have yet to be examined by the study authors. Of interest, women in the IMAGE program reported higher levels of communication with partners (Pronyk et al. 2008) and children (Phetla et al. 2008), potentially improving the way in which conflicts were resolved in the household. Additionally, access to microfinance significantly increased the value of assets in participant households (Pronyk et al. 2006), and qualitative data revealed that women's improved financial contributions to the household reduced marital stress and led to more harmonious household relationships (Kim et al. 2007). Finally, the community mobilization elements of IMAGE resulted in both individual and collective action around intimate partner violence in study communities, which may have reduced violence by participants as well as those in the broader study communities (Hatcher et al. 2011).

A second randomized trial focused on women's empowerment and health is Shaping the Health of Adolescents in Zimbabwe (SHAZ!). This program was designed to test the potential of a combined life-skills-education and economic-livelihood intervention on reducing HIV risks and other reproductive health outcomes among adolescent female orphans in Zimbabwe (Dunbar et al. 2010). After findings from a pilot study showed that microcredit actually increased health risks for female adolescents who were orphans, a modified version of SHAZ! was developed to better meet the needs of participants and included (1) vocational training with a micro grant; (2) skills building in the areas of reproductive health, HIV/AIDS, violence, and interpersonal communication; (3) social support through peer networks, psychosocial services, and guidance counseling; and (4) reproductive-health and HIV services.

This randomized controlled trial compared the effects of SHAZ! with a standard life-skills intervention. Initial findings showed improvements in economic factors and relationship power from baseline to follow-up among all participants. Interventions participants were significantly more likely to have equitable gender norms than were the standard life skills participants. Physical and sexual violence was reduced by more than half in the intervention group over the two-year period. Compared to the control group, participants in SHAZ! exhibited greater improvement in the areas of economic insecurity, experiences of violence, and low relationship power—all of which are thought to be important contextual factors that shape HIV risks.

As with the IMAGE program, what is less clear is exactly how participation in SHAZ! reduced participants' experiences of violence. SHAZ! programming did not involve male partners or efforts to directly change the attitudes and behaviors among the men in participants' lives, although its integrated social support component did include parent and guardian activities. The intervention and control group received identical information about identifying and avoiding spaces where violence is likely to occur, as well as self-defense skills and communication and relationship-negotiation skills. However, some aspects of the combined intervention appear to reduce participants' experiences of violence.

Several international studies suggest a similar reduction in violence resulting from participation in economic programs, although none of these involve either a randomized design or an emphasis on HIV. For example, Schuler and Hashemi (1994) found that participants in a credit program in Bangladesh were less likely to be beaten by male partners than women who did not participate in a credit program or than those who lived in villages where credit is not an option. Hashemi, Schuler, and Riley (1996) found that participation in a credit program was associated with a significant reduction in the incidence of violence against women. Qualitative data from several studies revealed similar themes, with women in credit programs reporting that their husbands hit them less often after participation, especially when loans came into the household (Hashemi, Schuler, & Riley 1996; Hays-Mitchell 1999; Kabeer 1998). A recent ethnographic study in India also found that the collective-action element that can result from women's group-based microenterprise programming can yield positive results in the area of reducing domestic violence (Sanyal 2014).

And notably, some scholars underscore that women's loan/lending groups may also offer group solidarity and identity outside of family ties. This is potentially important for HIV-risk reduction and antiviolence efforts, since some researchers see this form of social capital as an "associational mechanism" (bonds, social ties and social networks) that fosters critical thinking and reflection and serves as a catalyst for social change that can impact gender equality and health. Indeed, Larance (1998), Pronyk et al. (2008), and Sanyal (2009, 2014) all find evidence that social capital and associational mechanisms were important factors in shaping the ability of women to fight issues at the intersection of health and gender inequality (e.g., violence against women, male partners who drink excessive amounts of alcohol and then demand unsafe sex). Some feminist economists agree and think that the social solidarity that is produced in groups can be the basis upon which women can challenge constraining gender ideologies (Rankin 2002). While social-mobilization processes are powerful and appear to have great potential as catalysts for agency and social change, it is not clear whether this is the mechanism through which HIV/AIDS risks would be effectively reduced—or whether it is the economic element, or both (Pronyk et al. 2008).

Despite the promising aspects of these programs, several limitations of this type of women's empowerment intervention require further elaboration that are worth considering in the field of HIV prevention. First, it is clear that focusing on the need to empower women and girls while not focusing attention on men and boys can position women as being the parties who are charged with responsibility to change gender inequality and who must advocate for their own improvements in health. This can be problematic, because research has already shown that men generally have more structural and interpersonal power than do women, have more control over decision making, and strongly influence women's sexual and reproductive health decisions. Approaches that label women as disempowered and then ask women to take matters into their own hands—despite acknowledged structural and interpersonal inequalities between women and men—can fall short of desired individual-level empowerment and/or health outcomes over the long run.

Second, in chapter 2, I showed how it is limiting to conflate the notion of gender solely with women. Select scholars have instead pressed toward what is termed "relational analyses of gender" (Connell 1987; Dworkin et al. 2011; McKay 1997) or recognition of the ways in which not only women but also men are negatively impacted by the structure of the gender order at the regional and local level. Even in examples of best-practice gender-transformative programming, such as IMAGE and SHAZ!, men are only marginally involved in intervention work. Thus, while women are taught to re-envision the harmful aspects of gender relations within empowering health interventions, the very men who may partly shape the health risks in their lives may or may not be supportive of new gender norms.

Third, despite the positive examples that have been examined here, most women's empowerment programs that are in the evidence base do not focus on the structural drivers of behavior change. That is, even in these best-practice interventions, women in small groups are receiving either an individual or a group loan for economic empowerment. It is hoped that this will help women to individually negotiate safer sex. But scholars have pointed out that social structures enable and constrain individual- and group-level choices from the outset, and giving individual women the opportunity to earn some additional income may not be structural "enough"—because broader macro-economic trade policies, processes of globalization, and the ensuing local economic destabilization that has impacted numerous nations globally, including the United States, may be radically disempowering women on the ground, negatively affecting their health (Doyal 2002; Grabe, Dutt, & Dworkin 2014; Pfeiffer & Chapman 2010). Until the broader disempowering context in which individual decisions are made is reshaped, there is less likelihood that behavior change can be enacted or maintained. Indeed, maintenance of preventive behaviors is one of the key problems in HIV/AIDS-prevention programming, and there is some suggestion that structural and policy-level solutions can provide lasting effects for behavior change (Blankenship et al. 2006; Dworkin & Blankenship 2009; Gupta et al. 2008; Kim & Watts 2005).

Fourth, although many men are supportive of changing notions of masculinity and gender norms (Dworkin et al. 2012; Peacock 2003, 2013; Peacock & Levack 2004; Pulerwitz & Barker 2008; Pulerwitz, Martin, et al. 2010), some research has shown that some men respond negatively when they perceive that women are making societal and programmatic gains and they are not the recipients of these perceived or actual benefits (Barker & Schulte 2010; Dworkin et al. 2012; Dworkin, Hatcher, et al. 2013; Kimmel 1990). Men's responses to women's gains can lead to masculinism (the bolstering of all-male realms and the creation of new formal or informal social practices of exclusion towards women) and backlash (violence or other negative reactions), both of which can harm women's empowerment and health (these will be examined in depth in chapter 4). For example, female condom initiatives that focus on empowering women by providing them with a method "of their own" to protect themselves against HIV/STIs have revealed that some men react negatively because initiating female condoms can lead to perceived improvements in women's decision-making power or ownership and control over their bodies (Mantell et al. 2006).

To flesh out what I mean by this comment, I will cite a 2006 article that I coauthored with Joanne Mantell and colleagues at the Columbia University HIV Center for Clinical and Behavioral Studies, in which we argued that

[a] method that signifies a woman's control over her body may be viewed more generally as a sign of her sexual freedom, challenging male authority or overstepping local or regional values. In cultures where men control women's choices and opportunities, men may feel their decisions about reproductive and sexual health should supersede those of women. Some research suggests that men believe that use of female-initiated methods gives women too much power over sex, leading men to feel insecure or threatened. This may be especially pronounced in cultures where women's bodies and sexuality are viewed as literally belonging to the husband or where they are subjected to strong cultural edicts, such as female genital mutilation and wife inheritance/"cleansing" of widows. Thus, perceived shifts in gendered power relations brought about by the use of female-initiated HIV/STI prevention methods may not be welcomed by men. (Mantell et al. 2006, 2001)

In other words, during periods of shifting gender relations, possibilities for backlash may increase when women are targeted for empowerment approaches, given historical evidence that advances for women can be perceived as a loss of power for men (Kimmel 1996; Mantell, et al. 2006; Messner 1997). In the context of these changes, the initiation of female methods of HIV/STI protection can be threatening to some men, particularly if programmers and health practitioners exclude men and do not call for the introduction of this new technology into their relationships and bedrooms. To be clear, many men also embrace such changes (Mantell et al. 2006).

Research outside of the health realm shows similar backlash-oriented responses, at times, by men facing rapid changes in gender relations on account of women's empowerment. One study from Bangladesh revealed that domestic violence worsened from women's participation in a microcredit program (Rahman 1999). Other studies find the same (Mahmud 2003). In several of these instances, authors explain that microfinance/credit organizations sometimes inflict an intense pressure on women to repay loans. Repayment pressures can considerably increase household debt liability and can intensify marital conflict, a finding also reported by Hashemi, Schuler, and Riley (1996). At the same time, while some researchers find that improved mobility or social capital empower women, implying that programs may be protective against risk, just as many others find that improved mobility increases women's sexual risks through increased access to sexual partners, abuse, or sexual opportunities, an outcome seen in both the SHAZ! and other research (Dunbar et al. 2010; Hirsch et al. 2007). Indeed, the mixed findings indicate that simply accepting the simplistic assumptions in a sex-gender-sexuality triad (that biological women in heterosexual marriages are disempowered and can be empowered with a program that gives them resources to build their agency) without consideration of the social context and patterned gender relations on the ground and in households is problematic. This is particularly the case given that the social constitution of masculinity is highly dependent on the work arena and ideologies of providership and that several men report feeling threatened when their wives earn more income than they do or when they are newly economically destabilized (these themes will be examined further in chapter 4).

In 2010, my colleague and coauthor Suneeta Krishnan made this point by highlighting her own research in India, which found that married women who were unemployed at one study visit and began employment by the next visit had 80% greater odds of experiencing violence when compared to women who maintained their unemployed status. She also found that women whose husbands had stable employment at an earlier time point and then later had difficulty with employment had almost twice the odds of experiencing violence compared to women whose husbands maintained their stable employment (Krishnan et al. 2010). Krishnan concluded in another piece of work that "as gender relations shift and women assume increased economic responsibilities and decision-making power, the added stress of a perceived reduction in familial power may lead to forms of masculinity that are intended to protect men's privileged familial or social status" (Dworkin et al. 2011, 997).

Thus, in combination with the stressors associated with loss of income and entrenched poverty, a sense of destabilized power or authority for men can at times result in backlash in the form of intimate partner violence. This is not to say that we should not carry out women's empowerment programming but to emphasize that gender relations are relational between women and men. And, leaving men out of programming while attempting to empower women can have negative effects that can dampen positive empowerment outcomes, or can produce the opposite of the intended outcomes.

With this in mind, it is critical to point out that few studies attempt to examine the way men respond to women's economic empowerment, and no studies in HIV prevention have done so. Barker and Schulte's work (2010) is one of the few studies focused on men's responses to women's participation in economic programs, and they underscore that increases in women's income help men to see the value of women's participation in economic activities. In addition, in their work, they report that some men report becoming more supportive in the household because they are grateful that women are helping to relieve the pressure of the breadwinner role that men feel they are bearing. Third, some men adopted positive attitudes and helped to influence other men to accept women's economic contributions to the household. And finally, some men were already supportive of gender-related activism, and their partners' participation in women's economic-empowerment programming expanded this sense of men's support of women.

Simultaneously, however, Barker and Schulte (2010) also report that men whose female partners participate in economic-empowerment programs expect women to ask for permission to attend the trainings, thereby reinscribing inequitable gender relations at the household level. Other men demand that women give them the money that they earn in their enterprises. Some men reported that men's authority and household decision-making power are being undermined if women participate in economic-empowerment programs. Some men saw women's participation as threatening to male power, and hence conflicts increased in some households. Many men stated that they do not understand why programs are only in favor of women, not only in the economic-empowerment realm but also in their local contexts (e.g., where women's status is increasing or girls' education programs are being implemented). Finally, some men reported that they do not support gender equality trainings where men are not involved in awareness raising or sensitization meetings because they felt left out, confused, and suspicious of such activities. Thus, leaving men out of programming while offering gains only to women can alienate men at minimum—can negatively impact the outcomes associated with studies on women—or at worst can lead to various forms of backlash, violence being the most extreme example.

There are numerous other limitations of economic-empowerment programming that relies on microfinance and microenterprise to achieve health (or economic) outcomes. First, microfinance programs provide a very small amount of increased income to the households, and such increases are not likely to be large enough to empower women and restructure gendered power relations at the individual or household level. Several scholars argue that the word "empowerment" overstates the impact of microfinance and microenterprise. Venkata and Yamini (2010) find that participants in microenterprise programming were often found to borrow from many sources in order to meet the needs of their businesses and to pay off one source with another. Stewart et al. (2010) examined the impact of microcredit and microsavings on poor people in sub-Saharan Africa, examining four randomized trials and several case control studies. They found that some participants are made poorer by microcredit, given that they consume more instead of investing in businesses and that interest rates on the loans were so high that profits were not easily attainable. Numerous feminist scholars of globalization and development also argue that women are bearing the brunt of globalization, structural adjustment, and macro-economic policies and that programs place responsibility for economic health squarely onto women's own shoulders (Brett 2006; Goetz & Gupta 1996; Mayoux 1998, 2001; Sen & Grown 1988). Some scholars therefore believe that women are uncritically inserted into the logic of neoliberal markets through microfinance programs. These scholars critically assess the use of the term "empowerment" and claim that this sorely misses a broader understanding of how microfinance programs help prevent mass protests centered on the oppressive conditions that changing trade policies create in local markets.

In addition, it is critical to mention that in the past few years, there have been several systematic reevaluations of previous claims that microenterprise reduces poverty. This is important for HIV scholars because poverty reduction is one of the central mechanisms through which the empowerment of women is said to operate in microfinance and HIV-prevention programming. Specifically, two randomized trials and two reanalyses of previous studies were carried out in order to minimize individual selection bias (the fact that microenterprise participants are substantially different from nonparticipants in ways that are directly related to outcomes of interest, e.g., they are more well off or more self-motivated to begin with) or regional/community selection bias (the fact that microenterprise organizations actually select a region or community that may have a higher likelihood of repayment than more needy areas). Thus, the poverty-reduction effects of microenterprise programs have been vastly overstated globally, according to some scholars, including economists (Morduch 1999, 2000), and some argue that the poverty-reduction effects are limited partly because women are largely entering into female-dominated markets that are already oversaturated or that push women further into the private sphere (Ehlers & Main 1998; Al-Amin & Chowdhury 2008; Mayoux 1998).

Second, economic empowerment is only possible if women not only have access to resources but also can enjoy control over those resources. In my systematic review that I carried out for the Centers for Disease Control and CommonHealth Action (for the 2011 consultation mentioned above on microenterprise in the United States) (Dworkin & Hatcher 2012), we found that one of the most common findings in the global literature on microfinance is that women do not often have control over the additional resources that come into the household (Dupas & Robinson 2009; Goetz & Gupta 1996; Karim 2011). This raises questions about both the economic improvements that are claimed in these programs and the extent to which empowerment due to an economic mechanism may be overstated.

Third, gender inequality at the local level still shapes microfinance practices. There are gendered divisions of labor at home that pull time away from women's ability to be successful in their businesses (or restrict them to the home), and there are restrictions on their mobility in some regions of the world. There is also a lack of access to other key resources that would allow for further investment in businesses. And finally, it is critical to mention that there were some positive impacts on violence reduction in the IMAGE and SHAZ! programs, but there was less success concerning HIV-risk outcomes. The feminist and public-health hope that through these programs women could bolster their economic independence and reduce their dependence on men, which was thought to influence HIV risks, is possible but does not commonly result. Thus, such programs might be better described as providing small increases in income and helping in the survival of very poor households. Clearly, findings are very mixed in terms of "women's empowerment" (depending on how this is defined and measured) and in terms of the impacts that such programs have on women's violence and HIV risks. Assuming that working with women alone will bring about empowerment while not viewing gender relationally nor viewing programs as context specific and locally embedded can clearly yield limited results, whether the outcome being examined is economic, empowerment focused, or health related. This is to say not that empowerment is not possible through such programs but that it may be more limited to some forms of individual agency and may need to be integrated with more structural-level empowerment (agricultural livelihood and/ or property rights). If economic empowerment is a key mechanism through which to achieve better health outcomes, then might other economic-empowerment mechanisms be as important (jobs, regular work, access to and control over land, etc.)?

Working with Men for Gender Equality and Health

As was previously discussed in chapter 1, the idea of working with men in order to achieve gender equality emerged in the 1994 International Conference on Population and Development in Cairo (ICPD). The ICPD was crucial for movement toward gender equality in the field of global health and attempted to shift the emphasis in family planning from treating women in developing-country contexts as objects of population control who need to be made to have smaller families to affirming the need to "promote gender equality in all spheres of life, including family and community life" (United Nations Population Information Network 1994). It also focused on the role of men in accomplishing this aim. For example, the ICPD Program of Action documents state that

> [c]hanges in both men's and women's knowledge, attitudes and behavior are necessary conditions for achieving the harmonious partnership of men and women. Men play a key role in bringing about gender equality because in most societies, men exercise preponderant power in nearly every sphere of life, ranging from personal decisions regarding the size of families to the policy and program decisions taken at all levels of Government. The objective is to promote gender equality in all spheres of life, including family and community life, and to encourage and enable men to take responsibility for their sexual and reproductive behavior and their social and family roles. (United Nations Population Information Network 1994, 51)

While such a stance is clearly framed with certain assumptions about men's power and the pathologization of men's individual behaviors (instead of recognizing that gender relations are structured in ways that are harmful to men as well and that masculinity is not just an individual action but is shaped structurally, culturally, and institutionally), in the years that followed, for the first time the role of men in gender equality and health was included in numerous declarations and platforms for action. The ICPD stance has been crucial, and according to gender-justice scholars and activists, it paved the way for more work on gender relations and health and not just women's health. According to Peacock and colleagues (2009),

> Since ICPD, work with men for gender equality has gained widespread legitimacy and is increasingly seen as an indispensable means for achieving it. In addition to the push for equality in its own right, there is a growing recognition that dominant norms about manhood harm both women's and men's health. A rapidly expanding evidence base, described below, has demonstrated that rigorously implemented initiatives targeting men can lead to significant changes in social practices that affect the health of both sexes. (S119)

While it has been a positive development to see the increased emphasis in ICPD (1994) on "including men to take responsibility for their sexual and reproductive behavior" and their "social and family" roles and norms, it is the case that within the field of HIV prevention, "relatively few interventions explicitly attempted to address these norms and even fewer studies had measured the effects of such interventions" (Pulerwitz, Michaelis, et al. 2010, 283). Indeed, there has now been a shift from helping men to be more "responsible" and working with men as "partners" to improve women's health outcomes to programs that have been deemed "gender transformative" and focus on principles that recognize the costs of masculinity to men and women—and focus on gender equality. This is much more recent in the global realm and, as has been pointed out in chapter 1, this has not really occurred much at all domestically (Barker et al. 2007; Dworkin, Fullilove, & Peacock 2009; Dworkin et al. 2011; Verma et al. 2008).

Programs that emphasize work with men and are focused on the intersection of gender equality and health have generally been underpinned by two main frameworks concerning masculinities and health. First, there is recognition that men play a role in the perpetuation of gender inequality and that they can engage critically to reflect on this fact within groups and communities. Men are then pressed to act more "responsibly" in terms of family life, antiviolence endeavors, and their own sexual and reproductive health. This framing tends to ask men to be partners in improving women's health outcomes. While such an approach can be critiqued for a reliance on "responsibilization" talk, it attempts to engage men in the process of finding solutions instead of framing them solely as a problem.

The second framing of this work recognizes that when heterosexually active men undergo gender transformation (including a focus on promoting safe space for men to critically reflect on and prompt the emergence of new definitions of what it means to be a man) and work for gender equality, this can dramatically change relationships and communities to positively shape both women's and men's health. There is recognition that negative health effects can occur when men adhere to narrow and constraining aspects of masculinities not only for women but for men themselves (this is referred to by sociologists as the "costs of masculinity"). Here, researchers have underscored that when definitions of masculinities emphasize adventure (taking sexual opportunities no matter what the cost), risk taking, multiple partners, and inequitable attitudes towards women, these are associated with men's and women's HIV risks (Jewkes & Morrell 2010; Kalichman, Simbayi, & Cain et al. 2007; Kalichman et al. 2009; Morrell et al. 2013; Pulerwitz & Barker 2008; Pulerwitz, Michaelis, et al. 2010). In addition, recall material from chapter 1 that discussed that research has shown that men who are violent are more likely to be HIV positive than men who are not violent (Jewkes et al. 2011). Thus, there is a cost of adhering to narrow notions of what it means to be a man that impacts not just women but men too. Given this evidence, it may not be enough in HIV/AIDS-prevention programs to simply tell men that gender inequality harms women and ask them to be partners in women's health. This might partly leave masculinities intact and does not challenge men to reconfigure masculinities and the gender order. Rather, there is evidence that challenging current definitions of masculinity and focusing on the costs of masculinity to women and men can improve the health and attitudes of men and boys (Barker et al. 2010; Dworkin 2010; Dworkin et al. 2012; Pulerwitz, Michaelis, et al. 2010; Van den Berg et al. 2013).

Recall that in chapter 1 I laid out the conceptual difference between trait-based perspectives on masculinities such as "sex roles" and constructionist perspectives such as "masculine ideologies" in order to characterize men's adherence to norms of masculinity. Trait-based perspectives were said to be too fixed and too ahistorical, to link sex to gender uncritically, and to be based on the assumption that change resides in individuals. By way of contrast, constructionist perspectives saw masculinities as a set of ideologies that men tried to live up to as it was defined by societies, in local contexts, and in relationships with other people. Even though this was an advance over "sex roles," it still left room for improvement because narrow definitions of hegemonic masculinity that tended to reify some of the worst problems found in sex-role theory were deployed in the arenas of public and global health.

Just as a limited notion of a sex/gender order was applied to women in HIV/AIDS-prevention programming (the topic of chapter 2), similarly limited notions were applied to men in health programs. But thankfully, years later, several public health researchers thought that existing scales that were being drawn on in health programming—scales that relied on ideas related to "traditional masculinity," "sex roles," or "masculine ideology"—focused too much on men who adhere to current gender norms and did not adequately capture men who challenged those norms. In addition, several scholars state,

> [M]any of the scales that were created were not created with a focus on reproductive health, sexuality, or violence prevention and hence there was a need to develop a measure that more closely aligned with the ways that masculine ideals may be shaping these important domains (Pulerwitz & Barker, 2008). In addition, the existing scales focused on how men viewed themselves but not on how men viewed themselves in relationships with women or the extent to which men endorsed equality within their partnerships with women. Finally, existing scales tended to, particularly with an emphasis on sex roles, lack recognition that people change over time and that both individual and group-level norms can be modified. Thus, the "gender-equitable man" scale was born or the "GEM" to respond to these previous limitations. (Pulerwitz & Barker 2008)

Ultimately, the items that were created in the gender-equitable man scale view masculinities as constructed, as subject to change, and view positive change as men moving in the direction of more gender equality. The items in the GEM see a gender-equitable man as someone who, among other characteristics,

[s]eeks relationships with women based on equality, respect, and intimacy, rather than sexual conquest. This includes believing that men
and women have equal rights and that women have as much "right"
to sexual agency as do men.

[s]eeks to be involved in household chores and child care, meaning that
they support taking both financial and care-giving responsibility for
their children and household.

[a]ssumes some responsibility for sexually transmitted infection prevention and reproductive health in their relationships. This includes
taking the initiative to discuss reproductive health concerns with
their partner, using condoms, or assisting their partner in acquiring
or using a contraceptive method.

[i]s opposed to violence against women under all circumstances, even
those that are commonly used to justify violence (e.g. sexual infidelity).

[i]s opposed to homophobia and violence against homosexuals. (Pulerwitz & Barker 2008, 326)

According to the available literature, as predicted, the gender-equitable
man scale is associated with attitudes that men hold about gender norms,
and these attitudes can then be intervened upon to improve health outcomes. The GEM acts as some sociologists and feminists might think:
it is inversely related to men's history of physical violence and HIV risk.
That is, the men whose attitudes are the most inequitable towards women
are the men who are most likely to report that they had enacted violence against women in the past. The same types of trends held for sexual
and reproductive health outcomes. Men who were the most inequitable
reported less condom use with partners and less use of contraception
(Pulerwitz & Barker 2008). What these cross-sectional studies did was
set the field up for evaluations of gender-transformative health programming that seeks to move men in the direction of more gender equality
with the hope that this specific shift improves health outcomes. Several
interventions have been carried out with heterosexually active men in
developing-country contexts to see if there are changes between baseline
and follow-up on GEM and on health outcomes (and to see if it is specifically a change in GEM that yields the changes in health outcomes). Some
of these results are reported below and I offer readers some examples of
gender-transformative work with heterosexually active men.

The Promises of Gender-Transformative HIV Prevention Work with Men

Examples of HIV/AIDS and antiviolence programs attempting to reconstruct masculinities suggest that changes in gender attitudes and beliefs are not only possible but are successful in a large number of contexts. Many of these programs occur outside of the funded science base and within nongovernmental organizations. For example, the Men as Partners (MAP) program of the nongovernmental organization EngenderHealth was designed in 1996 to mobilize men to question the deep-seated patriarchal attitudes and beliefs that put the health of men, women, and children at risk. The program is implemented in more than fifteen countries in Africa, Asia, and Latin America. A longitudinal evaluation of MAP showed that participants were more likely than were nonparticipant counterparts to believe in equal rights for men and women and to express gender-equitable views about rape and intimate partner violence (White, Green, & Murphy 2003). The evaluation found that adolescent males were more willing than were older men to accept alternative views challenging the prevailing norms of masculinity.

As for science-based programs that draw on the gender-equitable man scale described in the preceding section in order to improve HIV outcomes, Program H in Brazil and its Indian adaptation (Yaari Dosti) have also been successful in transforming masculinities, violence, and HIV-related practices. Each relies on promoting more gender-equitable norms among men to improve both men's and women's health. In Brazil, groups of young men aged fourteen to twenty-five were targeted, and the validated gender-equitable man scale was used to determine program impact. At baseline, young men reported significant HIV/AIDS risks, and results show that agreement with inequitable norms was associated with HIV/AIDS risks. At follow-up, significantly fewer men agreed with gender-inequitable statements. In the intervention arm, there were significant improvements in condom use at last sexual intercourse with a primary partner. Additionally, in the intervention arm there was increased agreement with gender-equitable norms, and this was associated with reduced HIV/AIDS risks (Population Council 2006).

Within the implementation of the Indian adaptation of Program H, Yaari Dosti, the program resulted in somewhat similar results as did Program H at follow-up, except that there was a significant increase in condom use at last sexual intercourse with any type of partner among men participating in the Indian program. There were also significant reductions in self-reported violence against a female partner in the intervention arm in the Indian version of the program (Population Council 2006).

HIV- and violence-prevention programs that drew on GEM have also been implemented in Ethiopia. A quasi-experimental intervention with young men aged fifteen to twenty-four in youth clubs received either (1) a community-based program to promote gender equity and train young men to reduce HIV and violence risks; (2) a capacity-strengthening intervention that included technical assistance from the President's Emergency Plan for AIDS Relief (PEPFAR) NGO partners and service providers who focused on including men and gender in ongoing HIV work; or (3) a control condition. In both intervention arms, young men were less likely to support gender-inequitable norms at six-month follow-up in comparison to controls, and there were significant reductions in violence. Changes in GEM were associated with the changed health outcomes. There was limited change in reported sexual activity, however, because there were limited reports of sexual activity overall (Pulerwitz, Martin, et al. 2010).

Do Gender-Transformative HIV-Prevention Interventions with Heterosexually Active Men Really "Work"?

In addition to the promising results mentioned above, there have been several reviews to examine the efficacy of gender-transformative HIV- and violence-prevention interventions with heterosexually active men. Recall that in chapter 1, I defined gender-neutral, gender-sensitive, and gender-transformative programming according to the definitions provided by Geeta Rao Gupta (2001). These categories were innovatively applied to the available programs that work with men and boys to improve numerous health outcomes, including sexual and reproductive health outcomes such as violence and HIV risks. The point of applying the framework was to see whether programs that are gender neutral with men are just as effective as programs that are gender sensitive or gender transformative, or whether the latter programs are better than a gender-neutral approach in terms of achieving positive health outcomes with heterosexually active men.

In these reviews, Barker, Ricardo, & Nascimento (2007) and Barker et al. (2010) found that programs that were gender-sensitive or -transformative were more efficacious than those that were gender neutral in their content. These authors concluded that a gender-transformative approach that promotes gender-equitable relationships between women and men do actually work better than narrowly focused interventions that do not take gender relations into account.

To update this work, in my own systematic review with Sheri Lippman and Sara Treves-Kagan (2013), we analyzed more recent gender-transformative HIV- and violence-prevention interventions with heterosexually active men and found that nine of the eleven recent interventions reported statistically significant declines in at least one indicator of sexual risk. We also found that for outcomes related to violence against women, six out of eight interventions reported statistically significant declines in the perpetration of physical or sexual violence against women. And, in terms of challenging men to reconfigure gender roles to be more equitable and to reconsider what it means to be men, eleven out of twelve studies found some statistically significant change. In our review, we concluded that gender-transformative programming with heterosexually active men plays an important role in increasing sexually protective behaviors, changing gender norms to be more equitable, preventing violence, and reducing HIV.

The above findings largely reported on quantitative GEM or gender-norm scales and the impact that shifting men in the direction of more equitable attitudes and beliefs has on health outcomes. However, in chapter 4, I will analyze original data that I collected through an in-depth qualitative study of a women's rights–based and masculinities-focused gender-transformative HIV- and violence-prevention program. I carried this study out through a collaboration with the University of Cape Town and Sonke Gender Justice (a nongovernmental organization that works with men to challenge hegemonic norms of masculinity, reduce the spread and impact of HIV and AIDS, and reduce violence against both women and men). In chapter 4, I will closely examine how men narrate what it is like to be asked to change in the direction of more gender equality, particularly when one is marginalized by race and class status—and I will also examine the impact of the program on men's alcohol use, violence, and HIV-related behaviors.

Limitations of Work with Men to Reduce Violence and HIV Risks

Several limitations of gender-transformative approaches clearly exist. First, I and my colleagues Jenny Higgins and Susie Hoffman (Higgins, Hoffman, & Dworkin 2010) have previously argued that focusing on men to improve women's health can offer the impression that men are solely beneficiaries in a system of gender relations where they are being blamed for women's health outcomes. In addition, placing men at the helm to help reshape their own and women's health outcomes may reposition men as having control over decision making or may reinforce male dominance overall. Recall that earlier in this chapter, in the discussion of microfinance, I explained that some men wanted women to ask for permission to even participate in a women's empowerment program. If men are placed at the helm of decision making intended to improve women's and men's health, the question arises as to what this does to power relations between women and men—does this readvantage men relative to women? Finally, some researchers and practitioners worry that offering men information, skills, and resources with which to reconfigure gender relations while women's rates of violence and HIV are very high may shift much-needed resources to men when women's programs need more funding and attention. In short, some argue that a focus on men waters down "the cause" for women. (This will be covered below and in the next chapter.)

Second, there has been very little work that tries to understand precisely how men respond to health programs that ask them to change in the direction of more gender equality. This is a rather important point to underscore, because men in many settings may be losing social and/ or economic ground more generally, and then public- and global-health programmers are asking already destabilized men to give up power and privilege and support women's equality (often in the name of health). In addition, because gender is relational, it is not entirely clear whether working with men alone dislodges the gendered ideals that shape women's disempowerment because women are not the focus of this approach. And, many programs do not have follow-up times that are long enough to tell us whether changed men stay in a stance of more gender equality or whether they revert to more inequitable tendencies over time (Barker et al. 2010; Dworkin, Treves-Kagan, & Lippman 2013). Plus, even where men may embrace new forms of masculinity in both beliefs and social practices, we do not know if women are open to changes in gender relations or if they are resistant to such changes because of commonly held beliefs that men should retain household decision-making authority in numerous contexts (this is another reason why relational analysis of women and men at the same time is so important).

Third, these approaches often take societally produced norms of masculinities and then largely intervene at the individual or small-group level. It may be necessary to lift strategies up to the community level or to the structural level in order to shift norms at a broader level or change the contexts in which men's practices of risk occur (this will be covered in chapter 4). Small-group formats are costly and do not reach entire communities. Only three of the fifteen recent more rigorous interventions from our relatively new systematic review (Dworkin, Treves-Kagan, & Lippman 2013) included some aspects of community-level programming and community-mobilization activities to shift gender norms or improve health. In addition, despite the fact that chapter 2 has already underscored how sexual risks are shaped by the intersection of masculinities, poverty, and other structural factors, only one gender-transformative intervention with heterosexually active men addressed structural barriers to shifting gender norms and decreasing sexual risk and violence against women (Raj et al. 2013). Thus, despite the positive emphasis on HIV- and violence-prevention programs with men, this track of work has not intervened in men's structural disempowerment. Furthermore, given that scholars have argued vigorously that women's economic disempowerment relative to men is part of what shapes women's HIV risks, it is not clear how empowering men structurally would impact women's empowerment or their HIV or violence risks, and no program has been designed to structurally empower men while testing the health-related (or gender-equality-related) impacts of gender-transformative work on both women and men.

Fourth, there are a host of methodological problems with existing gender-transformative interventions. Very few programs involve randomized and longitudinal designs that do help us to ascertain change over time and do reduce the likelihood that individuals self-select into programs (the reason this is so important is that when individuals are not randomized into programs, it may be the characteristics of the individuals—and not of the program—that lead to the positive health outcomes). And, many of the studies failed to include comparison groups. There is clearly a need for more research in this area and for more rigorous study designs as well.

Fifth, none of these published studies (at least in terms of what material was included in the articles) took into account that there can be disjunctures between sexual acts and sexual identities among men who identify as heterosexual. Recall that this point took up a healthy section of chapter 2. Most studies on gender-transformative HIV- and violence-prevention interventions assumed that men who met criteria for being heterosexually identified were in fact 100% heterosexual in their actions. Researchers may not have asked about sexual partners other than female partners, or studies may have taken self-identification as the definitive category without considering the gap that can exist between sexual identity and sexual acts. This is particularly important because, as has been pointed out in chapter 2, masculinity intersects with race and class according to one's sexual practices. It is therefore possible that, in gender-transformative programming, men's risks were being reduced when they had sex with women but not when they had sex with men. We simply don't know much about the applicability of a gender-transformative program for men who have sex with men or with both women and men, but this would be a very worthwhile set of programs to develop and implement. This is the case particularly because homophobia-related items are embedded in the gender-equitable man scale and it would be possible to test whether shifts in homophobic beliefs contribute to shifts in health risks for men and their partners (and one could test to determine which partners experienced such shifts). The same could be said for biphobia and transphobia.

Finally, as one can tell by its name, a gender-transformative approach to masculinities and gender equality clearly privileges gender as the key axis for HIV- and violence-prevention work. This approach does not adequately take into account that there are differences and inequalities among men (Messner 1997) that shape health outcomes, and that certain men are more at risk than others of HIV, not only due to gender but also due to race, class, sexualities, and structural factors that have already been examined in chapters 1 and 2. By focusing quite a bit on the "costs of masculinity" to men (Messner 1997), rather than on the relational nature of gender or intersectional aspects of identities and inequalities, researchers miss an important opportunity for women and men to work together towards gender equality and improved health. Other critiques of and suggestions for future directions in gender-transformative HIV- and violence-prevention programming will be raised in the next chapter and in chapter 5.

Instead of continuing these lines of work solely along separate tracks, perhaps gender-transformative work could proceed by capitalizing on the strengths of women's empowerment programs while minimizing the negative inadvertent implications of the single-sex work that has been examined in this chapter. When I say this, I am not disagreeing with some scholars who have identified that "the value of all-male and all-female initiatives should not be discounted, because they fill a particular role in providing safe spaces for men and women to express worries, share their personal stories, and seek advice" (Pulerwitz, Michaelis, et al. 2010, 290). Rather, my call is to attempt to increasingly integrate women and men as active collaborators in future interventions, which is also acknowledged as being an important strategy for fostering equality and support among women and men (just as collaborations/coalitions with Whites are important for people of color and coalitions with heterosexuals are important for the GLBT community).

A relational approach to gender relations would also mean including women in programs in which men are reconfiguring notions of masculinities to fight for gender equality and improved health. While this may sound hard to understand at first glance for some readers (some argue that men may not talk freely in front of women or that men dominate public dynamics and women may therefore be reluctant to speak), as I will argue in the next chapter, Sonke Gender Justice and others have moved in the direction of women and men working side by side in their gender-transformative health-related work. In my conversations with the cofounder and executive director of Sonke Gender Justice, Dean Peacock, he reported that men do talk freely in front of women in their programs. In my own work visits to Cape Town, South Africa, Sonke Gender Justice staff also reported that the inclusion of women in programs can aid in holding men accountable for their public statements and claims about gender equality. This is important because men's public statements can, at times, be accurate, but can also, at times, be based on perceptions or misunderstandings instead of accurate realities that are occurring on the ground. In addition, it is critical to have men and women working side by side on these issues because both women and men are impacted by violence and HIV risks that are specifically gender related. Thus, it is not just important to help men be aware of gender inequality and its influence on women's health—it is also critical to discuss how the costs of masculinities implicate men in the gender order. This helps to challenge both women and men to understand how both would benefit from reshaping the gender order in a more equitable direction. Having men communicate about these issues with women present can also help women to understand that men do not simply benefit from the gender order but are also harmed by it.

In order to more fully understand the benefit of focusing simultaneously on how gender inequality is harmful to women and their health, on the costs of masculinity to men, and on how gender relations impact men's health, it is time to turn to a gender-transformative health program in South Africa that is grounded in women's rights, is masculinities-focused, and works with heterosexually active men to reduce violence and HIV risks among both women and men. The chapter will begin with background information about the South African context and the HIV/AIDS epidemic in South Africa. The chapter then moves into qualitative empirical research that was carried out to examine the impacts of One Man Can, a program designed to reduce violence and HIV risks for heterosexually active men. The program is designed and implemented by Sonke Gender Justice, a nongovernmental organization in South Africa.

4

"One Man Can"

A Women's Rights and Masculinities-Focused Gender-Transformative HIV and Antiviolence Program in South Africa

South Africa is located near Namibia, Zimbabwe, and Botswana (to the north) and Mozambique and Swaziland (to the east). South Africa has a population of approximately fifty-two million people, placing it into the top twenty-five most populous nations. Most of the nation's population consists of Black South Africans (79%), with Whites and "coloureds" both constituting 8.9% of the population each ("coloured" is the official term for a racial category in South Africa referring to mixed-race individuals), and Asians comprising 2.5% of the population (the remaining .5% is categorized as "other"). Women make up approximately 52% of the population, and there are many youth—one-third of the nation is below the age of eighteen. There are eleven official languages spoken in South Africa, and the new constitution, which is one of the most progressive, officially grants equal status to all languages.

Despite the fact that South Africa is known as a middle-income country and has a great degree of wealth (some major industries include agriculture, mining, manufacturing, oil and gas, tourism, and financial services) there is an extremely high unemployment rate. Unemployment rates are among the highest in the world and reached 29% in 2001, 23% in 2008, and 25% in 2013 (Statistics South Africa 2013). Unemployment is highly racialized and gendered. Black South Africans experienced unemployment rates in 2012 that were five times higher than those of Whites overall (29.1% vs. 6.1%) (Laing 2012). In the 2012 census, it was reported that the income level of White South Africans was six times higher than that of Black South Africans. Almost twice as many women are unemployed as men, and Black South African women experience the most exacerbated rates of unemployment of all. The highest unemployment rates are in Limpopo and Eastern Cape, the two provinces that are the focus of the empirical work examined in this chapter.

South Africa is home to the worst HIV epidemic in the world and has the highest number of people living with HIV (approximately six million people). There have been an enormous number of articles and books written to explain why the HIV epidemic was so explosive in South Africa. I refer readers to scholars such as Heins Marais (2005), Shula Marks (2002), Helen Epstein (2008), Mark Hunter (2007), Walker, Reid, and Cornell (2004), Debra Posel (2008), and numerous others who provide an extensive history on this topic. These authors examine how it could be possible that the prevalence rate was less than 1% in 1990 and then exploded to almost 30% among women in antenatal clinics by the year 2004. Because it is beyond the scope of the current work and has already been extensively examined, interested readers should look elsewhere to explore the ways in which these and other authors provide coverage of the social and historical conditions that shape the form and trajectory of the HIV/AIDS epidemic in South Africa.

Previous research has also already tackled how the spread of HIV in this nation is linked to racism, sexism, classism, apartheid, and circular migration movements between rural and urban areas and informal settlements (Hunter 2007; Lurie 2000; Marks 2002; Richter & Morrell 2006; Walker 2005). That is therefore not the focus of this chapter, and readers are referred to these other works. However, in this chapter I do briefly cover some of the factors that contributed to an exacerbated HIV/AIDS epidemic so as to familiarize readers with some of the key trends. In these works, researchers make it clear that an understanding of the epidemic would just not be possible without an examination of "the circuits and terms on which power, authority, value and opportunity are distributed—highly unequally in the case of South Africa" (Marais 2005, 10). Under an apartheid regime that strictly separated out African, White, Indian, and colored populations and drew upon forced and often violent removals, over three million people experienced removal from their homes and watched their families and communities become torn apart, destabilized, and/or killed. Blacks were deprived of their citizenship in 1970 and were treated almost as foreign migrants on their own national soil. And, the government subjected Blacks, coloreds, and Indians/Asians to extreme segregation in the educational system, housing, medical care, and even on beaches.

Many individuals think that things radically improved for South Africans after the mid-1980s, when the apartheid regime began to lose its grip on power, but numerous scholars underscore that social and physical dislocation, migratory flows, and poverty were highly accentuated by race and class when apartheid formally disintegrated (Bond 2000; Marks 2002; Marais 1998, 2005). Unemployment rates and income inequality in the late apartheid and early postapartheid period rose dramatically due to forces such as globalization, including market liberalization and privatization (Bond 2000). Some argue that in this time period, there was a collapse of formal employment, leading to very low marriage rates due to increasing economic insecurities, and women were being drawn into low-wage service-sector labor (Morrell 2002; Hunter 2007). In addition, much has been written about how population movements from rural areas into informal settlements (shacklands), and urban areas in particular, led to deep impoverishment and major health problems, and it is no surprise that these same areas experience some of the highest levels of HIV infection in the nation (Marais 2005). Simultaneously, however, it is important to recall that some South African scholars argue that the sociopolitical realities of South Africa are not currently a simple package of neoliberal tendencies, but rather an "active cocktail" of rights-based talk, free market capitalism, individualization, and communitarianism in policies (Robins 2008a). The structural changes mentioned above, which involve the intersection of race, class, and gender, provide an important context that will help readers to understand not only the gender-related vulnerabilities to HIV that exist in South Africa but also why some men who participate in HIV- and violence-prevention interventions perceive that they are disempowered relative to women (a sentiment examined in the empirical portion of this chapter).

As for the HIV/AIDS epidemic itself, in historical and contemporary terms, it is highly racialized, classed, and gendered, with the majority of infected people being Black South African women and the majority of people with HIV in South Africa living in poverty. A 2011 national-prevalence survey of HIV revealed a prevalence rate of 31.4% among Black South Africans, 8.8% among Asians, 7.6% among colored individuals, and 1.1% among Whites (Department of Health, South Africa 2012). The rate of HIV/AIDS among women is higher than among men, with a large gap between young women and young men in particular.

Approximately 7.6% of young men in the fifteen- to twenty-four-year age group are infected while 24.5% of young women are HIV infected (UNAIDS 2008). Among Black South African men (the focus of this chapter) between the ages of twenty-five and forty-nine, HIV prevalence was 24% in the 2007 prevalence survey (Shisana & Simbayi 2008). Much attention has been devoted in the HIV literature in South Africa to the gendered dynamics of infection, including uneven gendered power relations in sexual decision making, the linkages between violence and HIV/AIDS, and the role of poverty, economic dependencies, migration, and partner concurrency in shaping HIV risks (Dunkle et al. 2004, 2006; Epstein 2008; Harrison et al. 2006; Lurie et al., "The Impact" 2003; Lurie et al., "Who Infects Women?" 2003; Jewkes, Levin, & Pennn-Kekana 2003; Kim & Watts 2005; Pronyk et al. 2005, 2006, 2008).

As I described in chapters 1 and 3, violence and HIV are synergistic epidemics, and South Africa not only suffers from the worst HIV epidemic globally, but it has also been deemed one of the most violent societies in the world. Before I move on, it is important to point out that there are some legitimate criticisms to launch at this last point, including that it can be viewed as trite or insensitive or can even be seen as racist, objectifying, or too sweeping. This is the case because such statements can be read as potentially essentializing South African men or populations on the African continent more generally and negating the multiplicities of men and the complex social forces that shape violence and HIV risk behaviors. At the same time, the level of violence and repression that the state imposed on majority populations (Whites are the minority) was extreme, and current enactments of violence cannot be understood without an adequate understanding of colonial violence, apartheid violence, resistance violence, repressive policing, and social and economic disadvantage. Readers who are interested in learning more about the links between historical and contemporary forms of violence can turn to published work on this topic to understand it further (Altbeker 2007; Jewkes & Morrell 2010; Loren & Misago 2009; Kynoch 2005; Morrell 2001).

In contemporary terms, scholars within South Africa underscore that the murder rate in South Africa is among the highest on the planet, and while the majority of victims are men, the female homicide rate is six times higher than the global rate, and half of women who are killed are killed by their male partner (Morrell, Jewkes, & Lindegger 2012). South Africa is also said to have one of the highest domestic- and sexual-violence rates in the world (Dunkle et al. 2004, 2006; Jewkes et al. 2010, 2011). Violence and sexual violence against women are said to be near endemic (Dunkle et al. 2006; Jewkes, Levin, & Penn-Kekana 2003). National surveys internal to the country show that between 30% and 50% of men in this region are physically violent towards a partner (Kalichman et al. 2009; Morrell & Jewkes 2011), and in survey work, also internal to the country, one-third of men report raping a woman in their lifetime (Morrell, Jewkes, & Lindegger 2012; Jewkes et al. 2011). As has already been highlighted in chapter 2, women who experienced physical and sexual abuse at the hands of their male partners are several times more likely to become infected with HIV than women who were not abused (Jewkes, Dunkle et al. 2006; Jewkes et al. 2010, 2011), and men who have been violent and/or have perpetrated sexual assault are more likely to be HIV infected themselves (Kalichman et al. 2009). Research even finds that nearly one in seven women who have acquired HIV would not have been infected if the woman had not been subject to gender-based violence (UNAIDS 2011). As I will argue, this is not a statement on any kind of essential "African masculinity" but reflects vast and complex societal shifts that have helped to exacerbate the synergistic epidemics of violence and HIV.

Research attention within the violence and HIV epidemics in South Africa has not only been given to women but has also focused on men, masculinities, gender relations, sexualities, and HIV risk. Again, because previous scholars have already amply explored it, I will make only brief mention of this background work. Scholars have examined the ways in which apartheid and racial inequalities, industrialization, poverty, violence, circular migration movements, gendered power inequalities, and male entitlement, power, and privileges have interacted to produce HIV risk for men and women. Research in South/southern Africa has found that idealized versions of masculinity emphasize the importance of "control (unemotionality), physicality and toughness, competition, success, (hetero) sexuality and responsibility" (Luyt 2012, 35). Men are expected to demonstrate heterosexual success, with male sexuality often centered on penetration and conquest (Morrell 1998; Simpson 2005). Many men are socialized to display emotional detachment and emotional strength through a lack of vulnerability about emotions, self-reliance, and feelings of responsibility for providing financially for female partners and family members (Jewkes & Morrell 2010; Luyt 2003). According to the norms and practices of hegemonic masculinity, physical strength is often used as a marker for toughness, and violence is legitimized as an appropriate way to demonstrate power over others—both women and men included (Jewkes & Morrell 2010; Morrell, Jewkes, & Lindegger 2012; Peacock 2013).

Indeed, for many public health researchers, it is all too easy (and flawed) to pin the HIV epidemic on some sort of natural or essentialized African masculinity wherein men are viewed as having many sexual partners, denying women their sexual rights, and enacting violence towards partners with impunity. To the contrary, South African researchers who have focused on masculinities have argued that there is not one masculinity but rather masculinities in the plural—there are hegemonic and subordinated masculinities that are embedded in histories of colonialism and violence, apartheid, the transition from the official end of apartheid to an emergent democracy, and beyond (for more on these details, see Morrell 2001; Morrell, Jewkes, & Lindegger 2012). Thus, masculinities are not fixed or inherent but are fluid and collective identities that are historically shaped and changed, and as such, masculinities are not practiced in a deterministic or singular way but are fraught with contradictions, fissures, and, of course, differences and inequalities among men (Messner 1997; Morrell 1998, 2001, 2002).

The literature in South Africa helps us to understand why masculinities are constructed as they are and why men respond the way they do to shifting gender and sexuality relations. There is not just a gendered shape to sexualities, but there is also "a race shape of apartheid sexualities, and thus of anti-apartheid and post-apartheid sexualities" (Ratele 2009, 290). Here too I refer readers to other scholars who have underscored in a nuanced fashion how colonialism and apartheid, globalization and structural adjustment, poverty, gender, race, and class relations shape the collective and local practice of masculinities and sexualities (Delius & Glaser 2002; Hunter 2005; Morrell 1998, 2002; Richter & Morrell 2006). In particular, concurrency (the practice of having more than one sexual partner) is common in South Africa, but far from being natural or an essential male trait, this trend has complex historical roots that are found in high levels of unemployment and migration movements, the demise of the homestead economy, and the crisis in the affordability of marriage. Thus, having multiple sexual partners in contemporary terms constitutes men as highly masculine when they otherwise feel that they cannot set up or provide for a household and thus lack access to the attainment of a highly valued marker of masculinity in family life (Epstein 2008; Hunter 2005; Morrell 1998, 2002; Richter & Morrell 2006).

As I've described elsewhere in this book, South African scholar Robert Morrell has argued that hegemonic masculinity all too often is equated with male hegemony and dominance, which is erroneously characterized in public health as individual expressions of extreme violence, heavy drinking, sexual conquest, and risk taking. He calls for analyses that allow for nuanced recognition of the ways in which hegemonic and subordinated masculinities are shaped. He also calls for analyses of positive masculinities and shifting notions of what it means to be a man in a context that is already undergoing rapid gender transformation. Indeed, men are not a homogenous group and are already responding to social and economic transformations that are shifting not only femininities but also masculinities. However, only some analyses recognize that men in South Africa are involved and caring fathers, partners, lovers, and community members who are increasingly sharing power and are joining social movements to reduce violence and prevent the spread and impact of HIV (Dworkin, Hatcher et al. 2013; Montgomery et al. 2006; Morrell & Jewkes 2011; Morrell, Posel, & Devey 2003; Peacock 2013; Richter & Morrell 2006; Van den Berg et al. 2013), and the current chapter is part of this much-needed corrective.

In order to further describe the environment in which this gender-transformative intervention was implemented, I will present other important historical information. What do scholars mean when they say that South Africa has undergone numerous social and political transitions in the last several decades? As I pointed out in a *Gender & Society* article in Dworkin et al. (2012), some of these transitions include the official end of apartheid, a newly forming democracy, improvements in women's and children's rights, attempts to redress past workplace inequities, and resoundingly increased attention to the prevention, treatment, and mitigation of the HIV/AIDS pandemic (Marais 1998; Morrell 2002;

Naidoo & Kongolo 2004). Since 1994, South Africa has been characterized not only by changes in race relations but by rapidly shifting gender
and sexuality relations as well. South Africa as a society is viewed simultaneously as being rife with patriarchal authority structures across races,
ethnicities, and cultures, even in the postapartheid era, but also as undergoing massive shifts in gender relations and patriarchal understandings of power among an emerging regime of human rights and equality
(Hassim 1999, 2003; Robins 2008a, 2008b; Seidman 1999, 2003). And,
some argue that characterizations of men associated with patriarchy are
overdetermined, erasing differences among men across regions, locales,
and communities (Isike & Okeke-Uzodike 2008).

There is clear recognition that within postapartheid South Africa,
there are a multitude of legal changes and human rights instruments,
all of which attempt to guarantee the rights of women and children
(Hassim 1999; Robins 2008a; Seidman 2003; Walker 2005). While
race and class issues previously "dominated . . . politics during the
apartheid era, sexual and gender rights now compete for space in the
post-apartheid public sphere" (Robins 2008a, 145). Meer (2005) and
Seidman (1999) have argued that the successes concerning women's
rights were due to women who were involved in anti-apartheid efforts
and also pressed against oppressive gender relations. The challenges
for women in South Africa partly parallel Black women's efforts in
the civil rights movement in the United States to include feminist issues, including claims that their efforts would water down the focus
on racial equality and resistance from men (Meer 2005; Seidman
1999). However, because of Black women's leadership and success in
negotiating across different sectors of government and with a variety of social movement leaders, the newly democratic South Africa
had leadership that revealed a strong commitment to gender equality.
Facilitated by the 1996 constitution and the bill of rights, legal and
policy frameworks are now in place that recognize rape in marriage
as a criminal offense, require men to pay child support (and provide
penalties if they do not), seek to improve the status of girls' education,
provide harsher penalties for child abuse and domestic and sexual
violence against women, require women to be paid the same as men
for equal work, and obligate companies to hire women (Morrell 2002;
Posel 2004). Even in its first democratic parliament, South Africa had

the largest proportion of women in parliament in the world and has the most liberal abortion legislation available as well (Frenkel 2008; Seidman 1999).

While clear improvements have been made in gender relations in South African society over time, women are said to still constitute the most marginalized and disempowered segment of South African society. Women are less often employed in the formal sector than men, are less often formally educated, work longer hours for less pay than men (despite similar skill levels), and are disproportionately relegated to the informal labor market (Bentley 2004). Further, women not only constitute more of those in poverty, both in absolute and in proportional numbers, but also face deeper, longer, more severe poverty, while experiencing difficulties pulling themselves and their children out of poverty, partly due to a lack of access to land and job opportunities (Bentley 2004). Of course, these trends are different across groups of women. Of the overall population who live in poverty in South Africa, 72% live in rural areas. Of these, women comprise the majority. Rural women are still the poorest, least literate, and least educated group in the country. Female-headed households are on the increase, and these households are more prone to poverty than are male-headed households. Finally, women also carry out significantly more household and child-care labor than do men and carry out the large bulk of the labor associated with HIV/AIDS care (Peacock 2003; UNAIDS 2008).

Therefore, of course, there are challenges involved in translating rights and laws into practices of equality (we will see this in the empirical portion of the chapter). Numerous scholars report that while many constitutional guarantees for women's rights and equality are available, these can be met with lack of enforcement, lack of technical skill to implement, resistance, calls to reassert "respect for traditional culture," or even outright hostility, and this has meant that women do not necessarily easily enjoy their rights or freedom from gender oppression (Gawaya & Mukasa 2005; Meer 2005; Mubangizi 2012; Robins 2008a; Shefer et al. 2008; Sideris 2004).

South Africa's progressive constitution and emerging democracy has also meant the emergence of sexual rights for its citizens. In fact, in 1996, South Africa became the first country in the world to offer constitutional protection on the basis of sexual orientation (Gevisser & Cameron 1995;

Hoad 2005; Hoad, Martin, & Reid 2005). This historic achievement was "largely due to the ability of a male-dominated gay rights movement to form strategic alliances with the anti-apartheid struggle, to mobilize the master narrative of equality and non-discrimination and to lobby effectively during the constitution-making process" (Cock 2005, 188–89). Scholars underscore that recognition of gender equality and sexual rights as human rights was the result of "streams of identity-based activisms" working through the Women's National Coalition, which fought for women's sexual and reproductive rights, and the Coalition for Gay and Lesbian Equality, which had lobbied for antidiscrimination efforts (Gevisser & Cameron 1995; Hoad 2005; Hoad, Martin, & Reid 2005). As my colleague Amanda Swarr has stated in an article we coauthored about gender and sexual rights in South Africa, these "collaborations resulted in the integration of sexual orientation into the ethos of human rights during this transitional period. Simultaneously, a backlash against improving rights, combined with failed promises (economic, race, gender, sexuality, and rights-based) of the new South African government, contributed to significant increases in homophobic violence" (Dworkin, Swarr, & Cooky 2012, 47). Indeed, many South African scholars have argued that "there is a glaring gap . . . between the progressive character of official state, constitutional, and NGO endorsements of gender and sexuality on the one hand, and the deeply embedded ideas and practices that reproduce gender and sexuality on the other" (Robins 2008a, 145).

The enormity of the HIV epidemic has also stimulated scholarship focused on social movements on gender and sexuality relations and notions of health citizenship (Colvin, Robins, & Leavens 2010; Robins 2008a). Much has been written about the Treatment Action Campaign in particular, wherein citizen science, social mobilization, and new gendered and sexualized identities challenged the state, the health care system, business, intellectual property regimes, and the pharmaceutical industry. This was a catalyst for "the spread of new notions of health citizenship, sexual rights, and the democratization of science in post-apartheid South Africa" (Robins 2008a, 128). Concepts of "biological citizenship," which focus on the ways in which collective social movements mobilize individuals around health identities to demand rights, are used to describe the shifting ties among scientific knowledge, subjectivities, notions of identity, and political action (Lemke 2011; Nguyen 2005;

Petryna 2002; Rose & Novas 2005). Much of this work has focused on treatment-related issues and has been less focused on HIV prevention.

Similar to the points I made about the domestic epidemic in chapter 1, within the HIV-prevention science base in South Africa, there has largely been an assumed heterosexualization of the HIV epidemic in South Africa (Epprecht 2008; Jewkes & Morrell 2010; Maartens et al. 1997; Shefer & Foster 2009; UNAIDS 2012). Assumptions that the epidemic is largely "heterosexual" in South Africa mask the fact that many men and women might identify as heterosexual but have sex with men or both women and men (Reddy, Sandfort, & Rispel 2010). Indeed, while contemporary society is changing in terms of recognition of the contribution of same-sex sexuality to the epidemic, there is no doubt that homophobia has contributed to the absence of a full-scale response to marginalized sexualities—or men who identify as heterosexual but are not "100% heterosexual"—in the HIV epidemic (Reddy & Sandfort 2011).

Within a "heterosexualized epidemic," then, given recognition that gender relations concern the relational study of both women and men, and given that societal conceptions of both masculinity and femininity shape health outcomes for women and men (Courtenay 2000b, 2000c; Logan, Cole, & Leukefield 2002; O'Leary 2002; Sabo & Gordon 1995), it is clearly of central importance to examine masculinity. UNAIDS argues that "evidence informed programmes that forge norms of gender equity should be brought to scale, with particular attention to interventions focused on men and boys" (2008, 11). Morrell underscores that there are two solid reasons for studying gender and sexuality relations through the lens of masculinities. Similar to my points in chapter 1 is Morrell's argument that

[o]ne is to assist the move away from essentialism and sex-role theory which together promote analyses which rest on unproblematised and naturalised equations of men with particular traits or characteristics, including sexuality-related characteristics. The second, more important, reason is to extend the understanding of how gender is a feature of all social relationships which is part of a quest to understand how inequalities develop and are sustained and how power is wielded. (1998, 630)

To this, I would add that it is essential to intervene with men on the social nature of masculinities in order to create a safe space within which to critically reflect on the costs of masculinities, not only to women but also to men, to press for gender equality, and to improve both men's and women's health. An emphasis on not just the social and cultural privileges that men enjoy but also the costs to masculinity can help to reshape the norms and social structures that are constraining to both women and men and that shape their sexualities, and to positively influence health (Dworkin, Fullilove, & Peacock 2009; Dworkin et al. 2012; Dworkin, Hatcher et al. 2013; Van den Berg et al. 2013).

In the empirical work that comes next in this chapter, I ask several questions. Given that public- and global-health programming often asks men to change in the direction of more gender equality in order to reduce violence and HIV/AIDS risks in a context where men perceive that the protection and advancement of women's rights is improving, how do men respond to shifting gender relations? Do race- and class-marginalized men in global health programs simply embrace women's rights and/or gender equality, viewing this as a real pathway to improved health? Or are they resistant, offering masculinist and/or backlash responses and questioning the need for women's rights? Do men feel destabilized by race, class, and gender relations and calls for gender equality, perceiving that they are experiencing a loss of power or that their power and control are being undermined? Or do men welcome these changes as part of ongoing societal shifts that are underway in a still-transitioning democratic South Africa?

Several of these questions are answered through a brief examination of data that I collected with my colleagues and that was published in 2012 in the journal *Gender and Society* (Dworkin et al. 2012). The data was collected through focus groups in six high-seroprevalence provinces across South Africa and was analyzed in a collaboration between the University of California at San Francisco (UCSF, my home institution), the University of Cape Town (UCT), and Sonke Gender Justice (an NGO in South Africa that is dedicated to reducing violence against women, decreasing HIV risks for both women and men, and promoting more gender-equitable relationships). Examining these results is important because doing so provides a baseline understanding of where men's attitudes stand concerning contemporary gender relations in the regions in which Sonke Gender Justice implements its gender-transformative work (we don't have baseline data in the One Man Can Program because we studied the men postintervention only). Understanding how men view improvements in women's rights and status at baseline helps researchers to understand the promises and potential pitfalls of global-health programming that asks men to be more gender equitable in order to improve population health.

The remaining questions listed above can be answered through a second qualitative interview study that I carried out and that focuses on those men who have already participated in a masculinities- and rights-based gender-transformative antiviolence and HIV-prevention program known as "One Man Can." One Man Can was designed and implemented by Sonke Gender Justice in South Africa starting in 2006. It explicitly draws on the social justice legacy and civil society action and activism that exists in South Africa. The program developers and implementers of One Man Can view women's rights as central to the program and men as people who are concerned about domestic and sexual violence and who want to stop it. It sees men as people who can and do worry about the safety of girls and women and want to play a role in creating a safe, more equitable, and respectful society.

One Man Can sees men fundamentally as actors in a dynamic and engaged civil society sector and as agents of change in their homes and in their communities. The program calls for commitment and action by individuals and groups and provides space for critical reflections on masculinities and gender relations by pairing participatory workshops with community-action teams. The purpose of the community-action teams is for men to identify the issues that are most important in their communities and, when the workshop ends, to take up the issues of most importance (related to gender equality and health) through collective action. The reason why community-action teams were made an emphasis in the program is that its creators recognized that public-health-style workshops can have short-term impacts and need to be coupled with sustained community-level efforts that are embedded in local social realities and local solutions. The hope is that this coupling will result in longer-term changes that will positively advance gender equality and health outcomes.

The program content in the workshops is focused on gender and power (the way in which gender inequality leads to harm in women's health), women's rights, critical reflections on the norms and practices of hegemonic masculinity and their links to health, gender, and violence (violence against women, children, and other men), gender and HIV/AIDS, relationships (communication, respect, sharing power, decision making, and household labor and child care), and taking action for social change (at the community level). The workshops are facilitated by men and are held in groups of fifteen to twenty men. The sessions provide ample space for men to reflect upon human rights, women's rights, and how masculinities are defined, practiced, and can be challenged in relationships, households, and communities. The program has reached over twenty thousand people a year for the past several years and has expanded to North Sudan, Swaziland, Lesotho, Mozambique, Zambia, and Malawi.

In this study, I and my collaborators (Chris Colvin from the University of Cape Town, Abigail M. Hatcher, who was at UCSF at the time, and Dean Peacock, cofounder and executive director of Sonke Gender Justice) were interested in speaking to men who had already participated in this gender-transformative program (One Man Can). Here, we had numerous questions in mind: how do men view rapidly shifting gender relations and women's rights once they have had the opportunity to think about and critically reflect on these topics in the presence of other men? Do men articulate changes in their worldviews about what it means to be a man, and if so, do they attribute these changing points of view to local or regional shifts in South Africa, or to Sonke Gender Justice's programming in particular, or to something else altogether? What does a shift in the direction of more gender equality look like from men's point of view when it comes to embracing women's rights and/or gender equality? Do some men jump to accept gender equality once they have had the time to reflect on the topic critically, or do men struggle with, contest, and accept different aspects of women's rights, with some arenas feeling more acceptable and some less so or impossible to embrace? What happens when men try to translate abstract rights-based principles into concrete actions that are reflective of more gender-equitable notions of what it means to be a man—at home, in relationships, and in their communities? How do other women and men respond to them? Where men express that they experience sticking points or resistance, or when they embrace the gender-transformative program content, how can this social-science-related information inform and assist global- and public-health researchers to push men beyond viewing power as a zero-

sum game (where men see women "gaining" rights and power and assume that men therefore "lose")?

Finally, it is critical not just to examine the impact of gender-
transformative interventions on masculinities and gender relations but
also to understand the ways in which shifting masculinities and gender relations impact individual and collective practices linked to health.
Thus, in addition to asking how men respond to women's rights, I ask
(again for the men who have already participated in One Man Can),
what impact does this particular gender-transformative program have
on health-related outcomes? Do men articulate shifts in health practices
that are wholly unlinked to changing definitions of what it means to be
a man, or are men's stories of health-behavior change intertwined with
new configurations of masculine practice? Here, I am especially interested in alcohol use (which is significantly associated with violence and
HIV risks; see Kalichman, Simbayi, Kaufman, et al. 2007; Kalichman et
al. 2008; Kalichman 2010; Kalichman, Cain, & Simbayi 2011; Morojele
et al. 2006), violence against women, children, and other men, and HIV
risks. These questions will be answered through in-depth interview data
with sixty men that I collected in Limpopo and Eastern Cape, South Africa, in a collaboration among the University of Cape Town, Sonke Gender Justice, and the University of California at San Francisco. Men from
the local communities (Limpopo and Eastern Cape) who were external
to Sonke Gender Justice and who had experience researching gender
relations and sexuality studies were hired and were trained in qualitative
research methods for several days. The work was funded by a grant from
the Gladstone Institute of Virology and Immunology Center for AIDS
Research, P30-AI027763.

Now I turn to the questions focused on how men perceive shifting
gender relations that I raised a few pages ago. Here, I examine the results
from the 2012 article that I led in *Gender & Society*. This study involved
data collected through focus group methodology with seventy-eight
men across nine focus groups in six provinces of South Africa (Limpopo, Eastern Cape, Gauteng, Kwa-Zulu Natal, Mpumalanga, and Free
State). All participants were Black South African men given that this
particular population is disproportionately affected by the HIV epidemic and was the focus of preparatory work in the One Man Can program (Colvin 2011). The interview guide focused on questions about the

roles of women and men in South African society, perceptions of changing gender relations in South Africa, and masculinity-related beliefs and practices in families, relationships, and communities. Because this particular sample of men have not participated in a gender-transformative intervention that seeks to democratize relationships between women and men, we can expect that their points of view may not be as gender equitable as those of the men who have participated in such a program.

Gender Relations in the Occupational, Household, and Interpersonal Realms

All of the focus groups shared the common emphasis that the role of men was to economically provide for the family. At the same time, men expressed frustration at not being able to live up to this role. Given the literature examined earlier in the chapter on racism, apartheid, dramatic underemployment, and poverty in the postapartheid southern Africa context, it may not be surprising that the most common way in which men characterized changing gender relations was to emphasize that men were in dire need of jobs. They also had perceptions that employers were prioritizing the hiring of women over men. In turn, women's apparent rise into the occupational sector and into earning power was viewed as women's empowerment within the occupational structure. This economic empowerment was viewed as altering the ability of men to provide for women, reshaping notions of manhood away from men being providers and shifting relationship power to women's advantage. Many men described that they felt "useless" because they have not been able to live up to ideals of male providership, and stated that they have often come to be seen by their partners and children as not deserving of respect, particularly when they were not working.

Several men viewed changing gender roles and their own unemployment as a state of being relatively more disenfranchised than women, not only because women had recently been enjoying more occupational success but also because women can be supported by government grants that help to support households headed by women who have children. Thus, the fact that women had a source of income where men sometimes did not meant that men felt that their own decision-making authority held less weight in terms of negotiating household roles and in terms of authority over children. When women made more money than men, this was viewed as particularly threatening to the constitution of masculinity. And, while some men were getting used to changes associated with an increased number of women in the workplace, several men described that working under a woman was a struggle in the occupational structure, particularly if this meant taking orders from women. A few men across the focus groups disagreed and saw the trend of men working under women's leadership as an opportunity for gender relations to shift and for men to respect women at work.

Additionally, women were viewed as being able to increasingly secure their own material belongings, and hence older men thought that it would be harder to date women, particularly younger women, who increasingly had their own financial resources. Access to increased incomes for women were also perceived as increasing women's consumerism, which was perceived to increase the number of sexual partners that women pursued and to decrease the possibility that any one man could sexually or financially satisfy or meet the needs of any given woman. In addition to perceptions of women's improved access to the occupational structure and financial power, gender relations overall were described as explicitly shifting towards women's increasing relationship power.

Men also perceived that improvements in women's rights and broader changes in gender relations meant that women would no longer tolerate inequitable decision making within their relationships, and some men described women as becoming more vocal in relationships in terms of protesting against verbal or physical abuse and male infidelity. Overall, gender relations were viewed by many men as changing the way women's relationship power was structured relative to men, particularly among younger women. Additionally, given that men can face situations where women work and they do not, this structural change was viewed as reshaping the interpersonal realm where men reported that women made new requests to men for help in sharing household labor. While some men embraced the opportunity to contribute in new ways to gendered divisions of household labor, many men described feeling "feminized" by these requests. Several focus groups focused on the theme of men stating that that they felt "undermined" or "controlled" by requests to share household labor or child care—or by requests from women for men to more carefully pick their extramarital female partners. Only a few men disagreed with these comments, and these men viewed sharing household labor as part of a positive trend towards more equitable relationships. These few men mentioned that when women work and men don't, men can't expect to have the final say in all household decisions, and that it is helpful for men to contribute to household labor when women are working and they are not.

While women's integration into the occupational structure and improvements in income were very commonly mentioned as indications of shifting gender roles and relations, changes in the private sphere (requests for men to do household labor) and women's increased access to public spaces (community leadership) were other commonly mentioned themes. Men in focus groups differentiated being feminized at home from being masculinized in *shebeens* (taverns) and all-male drinking environments. However, some men disagreed that household labor is feminizing and criticized men who went out to drink with other men as not carrying out their family or provider responsibilities.

Some men underscored that a new trend of women's entrance into public spaces—and of coeducation—was a positive change in the community, and a positive way for women and men to learn about one another, fight inequality, and foster mutual respect: some men across groups said that they appreciated women's ideas in community meetings or groups and found them to be capable and compelling decision makers and leaders. In addition to men noting that women were making rapid entrée into the public sphere, many focus groups' discussions centered on the fact that women and children were enjoying some increased protection from the police and courts in terms of violence against women and children and in terms of child support payments to women.

Violence against Women

Numerous men in our focus groups also described how women seek the protection of laws and local, cultural and institutional enforcements when men carry out violence against women. Other focus groups agreed that the same was true not only for women but also for children. Some men mentioned their perceptions that women abuse men in the home, and stated that if they reported this to the police, it would not be taken seriously. Men frequently described resenting the way the court system protected women while asking men to pay child support, and many men felt that women's and children's rights were causing conflict and clashes in the home. Men often questioned whether women and children have a full understanding of their rights. Focus group participants frequently described a perceived destabilization of men's household authority given an improvement in women's and children's rights.

Overall, many different focus groups perceived that women were more empowered than men and that men were being degraded or diminished in terms of household authority and societal power as a result. Many focus groups agreed that male violence erupts over conflicts about women's rights, and many participants perceived that violence was increasing over time in South Africa—and that this was directly attributable to the advancement and protection of women's rights. Some men were clearly not opposed to women's and children's rights in the abstract, but at the same time did not approve of the specific "approach" that women took to requesting/fighting for their rights in relationships and households, perceiving that women were "too demanding." Here, men expressed a clear desire for women to present the case for rights less "forcefully." Other men explained that when women "realize" that they have rights, this was particularly problematic when women shifted their behaviors away from traditionally feminine tasks such as cooking and cleaning.

South African scholars argue that migrancy, unemployment, and racism in the pre- and postapartheid periods have provided a context that intersects with improvements in women's status and rights, resulting in a perceived loss of men's power. Here, scholars argue that men have adapted to feelings of disempowerment and alienation by seeking more sexual opportunities, enacting "hypermasculinity," engaging in violence, and detaching from family life to seek status in all-male contexts (Richter & Morrell 2006; Walker 2005; Wood & Jewkes 1997). On the other hand, some men have embraced change and have pressed forward with building gender-equitable responses (e.g., increasing their involvement in family and in HIV/AIDS care) and participating in broader social movements for antiviolence and HIV/AIDS prevention, alongside expressing firm commitments to equality and justice (Colvin 2011; Connell 1995a; Kimmel & Mosmiller 1992; Peacock & Levack 2004; Peacock, Khumalo, & McNab 2006). Still other researchers in South Africa reveal that men are responding to social and political shifts with spaces of reflection and criticism of past modes of masculinity without necessarily having a firm grounding concerning what kinds of masculinity will definitively replace or merge with past modes in the contemporary era—or form new modes altogether (Hunter 2005; Morrell 2002; Posel 2004; Robins 2008a; Walker 2005).

Indeed, these social science findings reveal that there are several critical points to engage with when carrying out HIV- and violence-prevention programs with men that seek to democratize relationships between women and men in the name of improved health. First, this data set includes men before they receive a gender-transformative intervention and largely reveals narratives that show resistance to shifting gender relations, offering masculinist and backlash narratives of improvements in women's rights. Overall, changes in South African society in terms of women's rights more broadly and in terms of occupational advances have led many men to feel that women have acquired new forms of agency and citizenship in South Africa while men perceive that they have experienced losses in the workplace, in relationships, and in households and communities (Dworkin et al. 2012). Some scholars argue that men in South Africa often find themselves "in the middle of what has been called a 'crisis in masculinity' in South Africa, a situation where liberalizing political discourses, the growing empowerment of women, and persistent levels of significant unemployment all contribute to a sense of uncertainty about the social roles and responsibilities for men" (Colvin, Robins, & Leavens 2010, 1185–86).

Naturally, pointing this out is not suggesting that it is appropriate for masculine crisis logic (i.e., that masculinity is being threatened or undermined) to be used for backlash purposes against women. Rather, it is important to underscore that while women are disproportionately in poverty and overrepresented among the poor, it is also true that rising inequalities and structural unemployment have made many women and men more economically and socially vulnerable over time. This has also made it very difficult for men to provide for their families, to pay *lobola* (monetary exchange a man makes to a bride's family), and to get married (Morrell, Jewkes, & Lindegger 2012; Robins 2008a). These structural changes provide an important context for men's feelings of disempowerment and destabilization, and it is important for global health programming to directly engage with these feelings rather than use a one-size-fits-all approach to gendered social change in the name of health. These results reveal the "tensions men experience when they confront the contradiction between embracing rights in the domestic arena and the widely held views that associate manhood with domination over women and children in the family" (Sideris 2004, 46). As we will see in the next chapter, however, this crisis also affords the opportunity for HIV-prevention and antiviolence programs to reframe masculinity in important ways.

Second and simultaneously, some men did embrace shifting gender relations—and thus, new formations of masculine identities that recognized and embraced more gender equality were clearly actively in the making. This is particularly important because citizens struggle to make sense of themselves within broader societal changes and an abundance of HIV programming that presses for "responsible, empowered, knowledgeable," healthy citizens (Robins 2008a, 164). In the concluding chapter, I will further consider the benefits and burdens of what this means as defined in gender-transformative programming.

Third, in this particular data set, it is clear that men frequently, but not always, viewed gender relations as a zero-sum game in which women gain and men lose. Hence, it may be important in HIV-prevention programming that asks men to change in the direction of more gender equality to link discussions of gender inequality with conversations about racial inequality. This kind of approach could honor intersectional understandings of the link between inequality and health and underscore the linkages between the need for women's empowerment and Black empowerment in South Africa and how both shape health outcomes. Drawing more powerfully on the history of racial oppression when discussing the need for gender equality can bolster men's critical awareness of the links between racial and gender inequalities when interventions on masculinities and health are attempted. Conversations with men could critically engage zero-sum-game thinking by including the ways in which Whites in South Africa and elsewhere frequently discuss reverse discrimination and disempowerment (or "special rights") when gains for marginalized groups are sought (Boonzaier & Spiegel 2008; Featherman, Hall, & Krislov 2009; Kimmel 1996, 2000; Knight 1994). This may engage men even further in critical reflections on masculinities and women's rights, as is suggested by multiracial feminists and critical race scholars who are focused on the intersectional nature of privilege and inequality, as was suggested in chapters 1, 2, and 3 (Bowleg 2012; Hill-Collins 1986, 1990, 2005; Thornton-Dill 1988; Thornton-Dill & Baca-Zinn 1984; Dworkin 2005; Higgins, Hoffman, & Dworkin 2010).

Fourth, this particular data set reveals the importance of talking with men in order to understand the contextual aspects of a given historical moment and locale that shape ideologies, beliefs, and social practice. As men are being asked to change in the direction of more gender equality in HIV- and violence-prevention programming, researchers and practitioners can engage more thoroughly and carefully with men in order to minimize backlash and harmful outcomes while garnering men's support for and enthusiasm about gender equality. As I will show in the next section of data analysis, taking on a more intersectional stance and bolstering men's understanding of the linkages between racial and gender inequality in programs may help men to become active agents of change in attempts to improve violence and HIV outcomes.

In the next section of this chapter, then, I evaluate the impact that One Man Can had on men's perceptions of shifting gender relations and women's rights. Before I move on to the impact that the program had specifically on men's views of gender relations and women's rights, it is critical to assess what men in this second sample thought to begin with about gender relations and women's rights in South African society. It is important to keep in mind that the men in this second sample may have not been much different from the men in the first sample (they were recruited in a similar fashion from the same partner organizations, and two of the six provinces overlapped across the two samples). However, the men in the second study here were subject to an intensive masculinities-based, gender-transformative intervention that engaged men on the importance of women's rights, challenged narrow and constraining definitions of masculinity, and linked gender and racial inequalities to negative health outcomes.

What I want to make clear before delving into the analysis is that it is critical in in-depth interview research not to sit down with participants and ask them how they have individually or collectively changed. There are a number of problems with this approach. It biases people to focus on narratives of change because of the way questions are phrased. And, this line of questioning invokes a lot of social-desirability biases (where people state that they changed or things changed because doing so represents themselves or their nation in a positive light). Making this the only line of inquiry in an interview guide would be to assume that the only way to talk about emergent social practices is through a narrative of change when it is certainly the case that change is not linear and that the very same people can both embrace and resist aspects of change (Pulerwitz, Michaels, et al. 2010). We were cognizant of these points, and we wanted to be attentive to these and rigorous about our work. I and my collaborators therefore found creative ways to ask about how societies and communities have already been in an emergent process of changing (and not changing) in the transition to a democratic South Africa—well before any program put its influence into the mix. We asked men to first speak about masculinities and gender relations more broadly before we asked men to talk about any perceived shifts in their communities, households, and relationships. And, of importance, we only attributed changes in gender ideologies and/or health to the One Man Can program where men specifically stated that they changed because of One Man Can. Not only did this help us to have confidence in the nuances of our findings, but it also led us to more deeply understand the relationship among individuals, communities, and broader societal shifts—all of which are critical to understanding collective agency and constraint that shape both gender ideologies and health practices (Kippax et al. 2013).

In order to understand how men respond to being asked to change in the direction of gender equality in gender-transformative health programs, it is critical to understand how men respond overall to broader changes in society concerning women's rights. Overall, many men in this second study described South African society as rapidly changing in ways that helped women to realize their rights. They frequently described the ways in which men embraced trends towards equality for women. For example, men like this interviewee from Limpopo reported that

> [w]omen's rights . . . not only in my community, but throughout the country is something that is said everywhere. Men now know that women have rights and that if they do not support them, they will easily face the music of law. The government does not take any nonsense when it comes to women's rights and that makes everyone change their attitude and respect the fact that women's rights are here to stay, forever. (Limpopo, age 36, married)

Other men agreed, stating, for example, "People are different but I would generally say that people are seeing the importance of women's rights. The message is being broadcast consistently on radios and television" (Eastern Cape, age 33, single). Older men in particular argued that inequality is something that should end, and they made explicit connections between racial inequalities and gender inequalities: "Women should be treated equal to men. There is no question about that. Women are equal citizens in this country and therefore they should not be oppressed. We were oppressed enough by the apartheid government and we cannot oppress our own women because we know how it feels to be treated as an inferior person" (Eastern Cape, age 51, married). While many men described that other men were accepting of trends that increasingly pressed for women's equal rights, several men were similar to those in our first sample, perceiving that women's rights "take away men's lives" and put power in the "hands of women." Such men viewed calls from the government for "50/50" levels of equality in the country to mean that "now men are victims and it has turned to '80/20'" (in women's favor). These men also perceived that their usual sources of gendered authority in households were being undermined, and men feared that with the advent of women's rights, women would stop respecting men, start controlling men, or, conversely, would stop needing them altogether: "Women are given powers to control us, through these women's rights. That makes them to not respect us any longer. They do not mind to go out and stay alone in their own yard so that they can just live their life without hearing from men" (Limpopo, age 56, single).

These narratives underscore a number of important points. The first few quotations reveal a perception that women's rights are being promoted "everywhere" and are increasingly accepted as a social norm that is promoted societally in media, policies, and the transition to democracy more broadly. Second is the recognition that within the context of legislative change and an active civil sector in South African society, women's rights were not a passing phase or an external imposition from the West but are "here to stay, forever." Third is the fact that several men articulated an intersectional understanding of oppression—that inequality leads to notions of inferiority and a lack of justice—and that such injustice means that men have an active role to play in reducing inequality. Fourth, for many men—even where they stated that they were at first resistant to the idea or practice of women's rights—the external pressure of the law pressed them to change their attitudes and social practices over time. In fact, men in our sample frequently made reference to and commented on specific policies that are drawn upon nationally and locally to help to achieve equality, using the term "50/50." This term conveyed the ANC's (the political party in leadership) stated goal of equal representation of women in parliament and the cabinet. And although the terms "women's rights" and "50/50" were often used together, and "50/50" was originally meant to describe the goal of gender equity in senior government positions, the term has come to be applied to a wide variety of contexts (household decision making, relationship power, and more).

Of interest, then, is the fact that many men in our study articulated that they were both witnessing and part of an already shifting terrain of gender relations in a transitioning South Africa. For example, similarly to the first study, men in the current study reported that in the occupational structure, "women are being promoted to high posts like school principals, circuit managers, curriculum advisors in schools. That means that men must report to them and we are seeing men doing their jobs and reporting to their women leaders." Many men stated that "most men have accepted that women can be leaders at work" and that this is "an impressive change" because "with women getting good job opportunities, men understand that they can be led by women, although some men take offense to being led by women at work." Unlike our first sample of men, these men reported that men experience "less pressure to be the sole provider" when women work, and that "women's rights are a relief to men." Beyond being viewed as a positive occurrence or an individual "relief," these trends were seen as part of the (fragile) transition to democracy in South Africa—and a boost in income for households where women worked. This theme was expressed clearly by a man who argued,

> I mean without women's rights, we would not say our country has changed, would we? Can you imagine a democratic country with men sitting on top of women and continuing to oppress women? It takes away respect for women and leads to a man continuing to carry the burden of running the show alone. Now that we have women's rights, my wife has a wonderful and respected job in the community. That means we have

a better income and we can do things better than when I was the only person bringing in an income to the family. (Limpopo, age 38, married)

Some men in our sample reported feeling threatened when women made more income than men and (similarly to our first sample) that "men at work are not changing" and "they do not want to be led by women." Additionally some men felt that other men "do not believe that women have constructive ideas" at work.

Several men reported that women's rights were critical not just to benefit women (financially, socially, personally) but also to build and develop South African communities more broadly so that they can reach their full potential:

> I agree that women's rights are a necessity in the community because it is part of community development. . . . [O]ne of the reasons that communities remain undeveloped is because women were not adding inputs into community development. But now look around our communities— women are driving beautiful cars and have built nice houses . . . they are running successful businesses and those businesses are contributing development to our communities. What I am saying is that women's rights do not just affect women themselves but it will help the community develop. (Limpopo, age 53, married)

Other men agreed that positive changes weren't visible just through the occupational sphere but in the community realm as well: "There is a change because in the olden days, women were not welcome in community meetings so they would hear about the proceedings from rumors. Presently women are welcome to fully participate in the meetings and some of them are members of different committees that we have in the community. These days we put women in first" (Eastern Cape, age 60, married). A few men felt that because women were being prioritized in several sectors of the public sphere, men were being left out—and that this was harmful to men:

> My view is that women have rights that have been given to them but they are abusing their rights. The present situation is that men are now subdued and women are trampling over them because of these rights.

For example, in church you will find only three men and the majority are women. Even in workshops [held in the community], women make up the majority and thus all decisions that are passed favor women because men are a minority. Men are naturally tough in nature and thus they do not come out to admit that they are being abused. (Eastern Cape, age 41, single)

Very few men described responding to women's improving status with backlash (such as violence), as was the case in our first sample, but a few men in this second sample did underscore that some men have a violent reaction to advances in women's rights. These same men often distinguished between "new men" who embrace gender equality and men from the "past" who were reluctant to change:

Men are violent against women as a direct action against equality. In some cases violence between women and men is about power. Men become powerless due to what the country calls for—change and equality. Some men will want to show women that they are powerful in a physical form. Some resort to sexual abuse and rape just to prove that they are more powerful than women and because they do not want to accept the changes. But in South Africa there is a new man. That man calls for equality. Gender equality. (Limpopo, age 30, single)

While most men spoke positively about the way broader shifts in South Africa led to positive improvements in women's rights and opportunities, I have already alluded in a brief way to the fact that men in our sample were acutely aware of how the law increasingly cracks down on men who commit violence against women in the home. Unlike the first sample of men, men in this second sample often reported this as a positive trend in South African society that was shaped by changes in the law and programs such as One Man Can:

I think the main positive change in South African society is that men can no longer abuse women. Our generation and our fathers' generations were guilty of abusing women. We did not see it as abuse, but as I listen to what the government and One Man Can says, I realise that it was some kind of abuse. I don't see women being beaten up as much anymore because the police will arrest you for that. Women have rights that protect them from being beaten up. (Eastern Cape, age 68, married)

Even where men partly accepted and partly rejected various aspects of women's rights, many men agreed that violence against women should not be tolerated: "Women's rights are for women. Men lose some power over women, but it helps that men must not abuse women" (Limpopo, age 41, married). A few men reported that while men may have cut back on the physical abuse of women because of the law, they would find other ways to abuse women, such as verbally: "The government has given women many rights—so much so that you cannot even shout at her. They now have more rights than us men. Now you can only beat her through your mouth because if you lay a hand on her then you are in deep trouble as you will be arrested" (Eastern Cape, age 28, single). Indeed, several men reported that the law "forced" men to respect and protect women's rights and that men would have been much slower to change without the strong push from the law and the criminal justice system. For example, one man reported that "like it or not," women's rights are being enforced by South African laws. Men in our sample appeared to be acutely aware of the possible strength of the law and often made remarks such as, "The police will lock you up immediately if they get that you are beating a woman." Some men reported that even where men had not previously accepted women's rights, the law has helped them to "learn to understand that we have to respect women and also give them a chance to grow in order for them to be better humans in the community" (Limpopo, age 31, single). Finally, some men in our sample underscored that the nation still has a long way to go in terms of preventing women's rights violations and said that they had been watching women get abused since they were children, expressing disappointment that this fragile democratic country had not come farther in this area.

While many men in our sample reported that men in South African society are coming to accept shifts in the direction of more gender equality, some men were more similar to our first sample of men, who offered great resistance to these changes. Many interviewees underscored that this resistance depended on age. For example, some men reported that young men are likely to change in terms of accepting shifting gender roles and women's rights but that older men "are difficult to change." At the same time, other men in our sample reported that older men are more flexible in their gender roles and open to new notions of masculinities and that young men were more rigid and disrespectful towards women (and other men). Each generation seemed to blame the other for rigid constructions of masculinity and for the subsequent negative health outcomes in South African society.

A few men reported that gender relations were worsening radically over time, reporting that because the law doesn't allow men to express themselves with violence openly, men are abusing women more secretly and privately—"doing it in hiding" (i.e., drinking at home and being violent at home)—instead of making a public "display" of their "big problems." These few narratives seemed to blame the introduction of women's rights into the home for increased violence, as was suggested above. Other men underscored that men will say one thing and do another when it comes to violence and the acceptance of women's rights—that is, there was a recognized disjuncture between discourse and action whereby some men publicly offered support for women's rights but "when they go in their homes, the opposite is the case." And, young men in particular expressed that they were quite disappointed that women's rights in the new South Africa meant that they could not "discipline" (i.e., physically abuse) their partners in cases of infidelity or where women "disrespected" or "humiliated" men: "It makes it even hard to argue or discipline your girlfriend because she will tell you that she has the right to walk with anybody or call anyone. We can't do anything to them because they tell us that they will report us to the police if we ever lay a hand on them" (Eastern Cape, age 21, single).

While younger men were more likely to express disappointment in what women's rights might mean in their relationships, they were also more likely to express that they experienced intense peer pressure to constitute masculinity as violence against women in front of other men:

> The popular view is that it is right to beat up your girlfriend. If you have never beaten her up for anything for up to two months then other boys will laugh at you and say that you are not man enough. They will tell you stories about seeing her with other men and if you still do not beat her up, you will be made the stupid person of the group. (Eastern Cape, age 17, single)

I will return at the end of the chapter to this point about men constituting masculinity through violence in the presence of other men.
Overall, however, thus far, these findings presented above have
focused on how men within a gender-transformative health program
viewed rapidly shifting gender relations and improvements in wom-
en's rights. These results are consistent with previous work outside of
the health realm that has been focused on men's reactions to women's
rights in South Africa and how men offer a mixture of support, masculinism, and backlash (Dworkin et al. 2012; Peacock, Khumale, &
McNab 2006; Posel 2004; Shefer et al. 2008; Walker 2005). As we will
see next, men who participated in One Man Can (OMC) reported
that their acceptance of gender equality was largely attributable to the
program, which, in turn, impacted the specificities of their attitudes
and social practices in relationships and households. In this next section, then, I describe the ways in which men specifically narrated how
their participation in OMC changed their view of gender relations,
and how this shifted their own enactments of relationship power and
of masculinity itself.

One Man Can (OMC) is a rights-based program that centers on engaging men in critical discussions of how social inequality operates and
how these social processes shape health outcomes. Thus, men who participated in OMC had the opportunity to think about the ways in which
marginalization operates to diminish and constrain certain populations,
such as the ways in which gender relations harm women and men and
negatively impact their health outcomes—and the way racial inequality operates and negatively impacts the health of Black South Africans.
Instead of negating human agency and possibly leading individuals and
communities to become immobilized by these inequalities, the program
worked to actively engage men in a process of individual-, relationship-,
and community-level change. The first theme that emerged from our
discussion with OMC participants was that many men in our sample
described how OMC helped them to have critical realizations about inequalities, pressing them to consider that, like all people, women were
valuable and challenging their previous ideas that femininity is equated
with subordination and inferiority: "I used to think that women are
inferior and will remain inferior. I then thought during and after the
workshops and realized that women's rights are an important element of

balancing what we took away from women for a very long time" (Limpopo, age 25, single). Several other men, like this one, agreed:

> There is a change that can be credited to the One Man Can training. . . .
> We, the older generation, grew up in disregard of women's rights. To us,
> women were supposed to be subservient to men, agree with men, and
> also know that men were the heads of the household. We did not know
> anything about women's rights. We have come to realize that women have
> to be treated as equals in the home and in the community and we are not
> supposed to abuse them. (Eastern Cape, age 62, single)

Many men also articulated critiques of patriarchal views of authority and decision making in households (where men tend to see their word as the final word in the household while treating women as if their points of view are irrelevant or don't matter). The shifts that were described were ultimately critiques of men's decision-making dominance in households, which facilitated viewing women as more visible:

> A lot has changed. . . . My childhood observations about man as boss
> were wrong. Before I attended One Man Can sessions, I continued to be-
> lieve the same wrong things that need to be done. But after some sessions
> and engagement in discussions with various people with various points of
> view, I then realized that it is wrong to treat women like they do not exist.
> (Limpopo, age 32, single)

What is interesting about the quotation above is that this is not at first glance a riveting account of gender equality. However, it is a complex narrative that delves into what a change in the direction of more gender equality looks like from the perspective of someone who had previously held a tight grip on patriarchal authority. Without giving up a hold on male-dominated decision-making power, it would be impossible to see and hear women's voices, needs, aspirations, or views. Thus, because OMC program content included the importance of shared decision-making power and open and respectful communication—and afforded men the opportunity to discuss this among other men—men shifted their view towards seeing women as having unique contributions, needs, and points of view. This is a critical step in moving in the direction of more gender equality, although of course this narrative indicates that this is a start of an otherwise long and complex process.

In addition to men articulating that the OMC workshops helped them to shift away from beliefs that women were inferior to men or didn't deserve visibility, men described an improved awareness of women's rights specifically derived from OMC. Prior to participating in OMC, many men saw women's rights as irrelevant to men:

> There are new things that I learned from One Man Can sessions. With women's rights, I always thought that it was a women's issue. It had nothing to do with men. I cared less about women's rights and more about how our parents had treated women. This was the only right thing to do, I convinced myself. But after attending Sonke's session on gender roles, I started seeing things differently and since then I fell in love with the topic. If I did not join OMC, I would still be stuck in wrong and degrading activities towards women. Thanks to OMC for opening my forever closed eyes. (Limpopo, age 42, married)

While some people reading this quotation might criticize this approach as one that "tells" men what is right to do in a health program, the program developers and implementers were quite clear that the role of the facilitators was not to tell men what to do. Rather, program facilitators helped to draw many men into the conversation, and the emergent social processes that resulted when men spoke openly with other men frequently led them to critically reflect upon the beliefs that they had once held dear. This approach is viewed as being more in line with consciousness raising, which respects the views of actors, honors the concept of agency, and has long been viewed as having positive impacts on the mobilization of social change (Freire 1993; Paiva 2002). In fact, several men in our sample described how men's position of power in households and communities had previously been accepted uncritically, but said that OMC sessions challenged them by highlighting how gendered privileges were actually a form of gender oppression and inequality:

> We grew up in an era of women's oppression. We admired and supported the way things were done. Men were the head and masters of the household and their pride was in that authority and control. The man's place

was the cattle *kraal* and, no matter how big the task was, would not help in any household activities as that was the domain of women. With these teachings from Sonke, I now realize that what we thought was good was in face a form of slavery to our mothers and wives. That was oppression at its best. (Eastern Cape, age 66, married)

Many men in our sample said to us that they would not have changed without OMC: "I would not have changed [without OMC]. I am sure that I would be sitting at home and expecting someone to do things for me. I have a great understanding of women's rights now and I have changed in terms of my perception of women in the community" (Limpopo, age 37, married).

Now on to the second theme. One of the most common questions that is put forward about programs that strive to "change" men in the direction of more gender equality is the question of how men will be convinced that they can benefit from gender equality and women's rights. Many people ask, wouldn't most men just assume that they have little to gain and a lot (of power, control, and decision-making authority) to lose if they embrace equality and women's rights? Wouldn't this particularly be the case for men who have experienced severe race and class marginalization and structural oppression? Here, Sonke's workshops were specifically focused on challenging the zero-sum logic that was so commonly articulated in our first study (where men think that if women gain, men therefore lose) in two ways. First, the program materials did not solely focus on the ways in which gender inequality harms women and their health, but the program also focused on the ways in which men are negatively impacted in the gender order when they adhere to narrow and constraining definitions of masculinity. In this way, men were less likely to feel "blamed" for gender inequality and were more likely to engage in a process of reflection that would lead to benefits for both women and men. Second, Sonke's OMC program content drew upon recognition of the strength of civil society (grassroots community action that involves actively engaged citizens) in South Africa, which, as I have pointed out, has enjoyed a long history of human rights activism. The workshops therefore emphasized how men can play an active and agentic role in improving women's rights—just as the oppression of Black South Africans could not have been (partly) lifted without the support of White South Africans. It may be no surprise then that men articulated that they saw how they could gain from embracing gender equality: "Honestly, I had a bad attitude about women's rights. I used to think that women's rights are about oppressing men. But most importantly, I have learnt through One Man Can discussions that women's rights cannot be realized without men's engagement to support the women" (Limpopo, age 36, married). Men articulated that prior to participation in OMC, they perceived that women's rights were focused on harming and oppressing men (taking away men's power and rights). After OMC sessions, however, men said that women's rights were not about taking rights away from men but that men had a role to play in supporting women's rights. Particularly in the area of intimate partner violence, men embraced women's rights and credited both changes in government policies and OMC workshops for their changed view. Men also articulated new levels of awareness of the role that men play in ending violence against women, and they viewed themselves as agentic in being proponents of women's rights:

> I personally must say that the workshop added to my interests on protecting women and children from being abused. It is through the workshops that I now know that women's rights will not be achieved without men's intervention because they are mostly the causes or they are the ones who abuse women. Women's rights are man made and men can turn it around or reverse it. (Limpopo, age 38, married)

While many men in our sample stated that OMC helped them to embrace women's rights, some men certainly described resistance, contestation, and ambivalence, even after OMC. These men, similarly to the men in our first study, still perceived that women's rights "take away" men's social power. When asked to share decision-making power with women, some men felt that a cherished source of gendered authority in households and relationships was being taken away. These men feared not only that women's rights meant that women would stop respecting men but also that women would start controlling men, or would even stop needing men at all. Finally, several men agreed with an emphasis on women's rights in principle or in the abstract, but in practice, they felt that the police and criminal justice system had "gone too far" because they were perceived as protecting only women from abuse (and not men). These narratives underscored that men saw themselves as also deserving unique rights and protections (and again, that women's rights have taken things too far):

> Women's rights protect women so much that now women do whatever they want to because they know that the law will protect them. If a woman reports that you did something wrong to her, the police will only listen to her story and they will just arrest you [the man] without listening to your side of the story. I am not saying it is a bad thing for women to have rights but I think women are abusing a good thing that was supposed to benefit them. (Eastern Cape, age 25, single)

The notion of women's abuse of rights and unfair treatment at the hands of police is a common narrative among men in South Africa (Colvin, Robins, & Leavens 2010; Dworkin et al. 2012) and may represent a growing cultural script about men's experiences of maltreatment by police and their general sense of being unable to influence the state to recognize and protect local social and cultural norms. This in turn often reflects a belief that many of the political changes since the end of apartheid have been shaped by ideologies "foreign" to local values and practices (for an in-depth examination of this point see Dworkin et al. 2012). It may also reflect many people's experiences of a police force that is increasingly perceived as unaccountable and disdainful in its treatment of ordinary citizens. Such narratives are also consistent with what other scholars have found when gender relations are rapidly shifting and men feel destabilized by these shifts (Kimmel 1990, 2000; Sideris 2004). These narratives are also not uncommon across other social locations—-e.g., where Whites think that minorities have taken their demands "too far" or heterosexuals argue that GLBT populations have pressed "their agenda" too far or are "putting their lifestyle in your face" too much (Featherman, Hall, & Krislov 2009; Kimmel 1996, 2000; Knight 1994).

A third theme in our data analysis that can be described very briefly and simply that I touched upon earlier in the results and when describing the OMC program is that many men underscored the importance of talking with other men to bolster their current understanding of and support for women's rights in practice:

I changed massively. The approach used was so good in a way . . . one has managed to hear other men's inputs and experiences. It is the inputs from other men and the experiences that made me gather more about what I knew about women's rights. I have clear knowledge now that women's rights is a force to be reckoned and if we as men do not help women to go closer to realizing their rights then women on their own may not. Women's rights are well achieved by the help of men . . . for women it is to know and understand but for men it is to practise women's rights. (Limpopo, age 38, married)

It is important to mention that the OMC program now includes both women and men in the same workshops because of the ways in which organizational leaders at Sonke Gender Justice view gender as relational (Connell 1987). These leaders find it important if not critical for women and men to work together in the struggle for gender equality and improved health. Because we did not carry out a comparative analysis of gender-transformative programs where we compared single groups of men to groups of women and men, we cannot comment further on the benefits of one over the other. However, despite the fears that exist that men will "take over" or dominate programs where women and men are side by side (reducing the potential health benefits that women experience), some HIV researchers have shown the opposite—that mixed-gender interventions have the same benefits for women as women-only programming (El-Bassel et al. 2003). But, researchers have not examined the benefits of male-only versus mixed-gender groups and have not compared health outcomes for these different groupings. This would be a fertile area for future research.

A fourth important theme within our current study was that participation in One Man Can led to changes in men's conceptions of masculinities and that this in turn impacted interpersonal decision making, contributions to household labor, and the exercise of gendered power in relationships. These narratives were often expressed through key descriptions of how men translated abstract concepts of rights and decision-making authority into practice with their own female partners and wives:

I used to think that women must listen to everything that men say, but now my wife says I have changed because I tell her when I want to do something, like buying something in the house—I ask her inputs. I used to come home and sit as she cooked, did laundry, and cleaned the house alone with the children, but now I cook for my daughters when they are busy cleaning or doing laundry or when they are studying. (Limpopo, age 41, married)

Other men agreed that changes in their own behavior in relationships were achieved by translating abstract concepts such as "women's rights" discussed in the workshops into practical action in the home and in relationships (e.g., "helping" with household labor):

I had heard about women's rights but did not fully understand what they meant. For an example, if you have a wife and a child you will find that the wife is cooking at the same time taking care of the child while the husband is watching TV. One Man Can made me realize that in such a situation, the man must also be helping her. I now know that household chores are not only for women but the man should also help. (Eastern Cape, age 25, single)

Here, it is clear that One Man Can engaged men in topics that reframed household roles and responsibilities as part of a healthy, respectful, and more equitable relationship. Thus, rather than approaching the problem solely from the perspective that women's rights is an abstract or normative position that details what men "ought to do" because the government states that it is the right thing to do, the workshops drew on men's views and actual life experiences to question social norms in practice. Questioning gendered roles in the context of men's experiences and having a chance to try new roles out at home (and to come back and talk about these) is an important strategy used in the workshops. This strategy was particularly effective, it seemed, in encouraging men to challenge their notions of power, respect, and dominance:

At the training we were advised on how to treat our girlfriends and about the importance of treating them well. That training made a difference to me because I liked what was being said there so I decided to apply it to my own life and I am seeing a difference in the way I am treating my girlfriend. (Eastern Cape, age 23, single)

A few men explained to us that men are in a position to listen more to their partners and change their notions of what it means to be a man not because of One Man Can but because of the way in which women have enjoyed improved rights and economic well-being in South Africa:

> Since democracy in South Africa, I have seen most men I know changing the way things are done in their homes. It is clear that because women have powers to go out and look for jobs, men understand that they also have a voice on how to manage families. Sometimes then, men used to be the ones who will go out and fend for the family. Today even women are able to go out and fend. Sometimes a woman goes out while the man is left home without work. As a result, men are in a position to listen to their women's views. Men today have changed from feeling that they are more powerful and thinking that they think better than women. They understand that women have inputs into family decisions. Decisions like where should their children attend school, methods of saving money, and how money should be used. This also includes understanding that when women are not ready or not in a mood for sex is fine until she is ready. (Limpopo, age 42, married)

Overall, men in our sample, however, often attributed their changes in beliefs and social practices to participation in OMC. They described a shift from male-dominated decision making, including a willingness to demand that their partners have sex with them, to a more consultative approach to relationships:

> Before I joined One Man Can, I was very critical of women's rights, or more accurately, I did not believe there was any need for women to be accorded special rights. In one of my frequent drunken states, I would go and look for my girlfriend, and when I wanted her to come along there would be no compromise. My word was the final word and I would not take any input from her. Attending the One Man Can workshops, I got to understand the wrongs of my past behavior and I started understanding that men should also listen to women's input. (Eastern Cape, age 33, single)

Readers can now probably see that the data is beginning to move away from showing changes in ideologies about gender relations and is moving towards showing how specific shifts in these ideologies may have influenced health outcomes (here, alcohol use). Therefore, it is time to switch to the final empirical portion of the chapter, which examines the way that One Man Can impacted men's health practices (alcohol use, safer sex, violence) at the individual and community level. The most commonly articulated change in health practices that was attributed to One Man Can in our sample was men's reduction in alcohol use. One-third of the men in our sample reported a reduction in alcohol intake after participating in OMC. This is particularly important given that research shows that it is reductions in volume rather than reductions in frequency of alcohol intake that predict reductions in sexual risks (Kalichman, Simbayi, Kaufman, et al. 2007). One of the most prominent themes in our study is that many men's reductions in alcohol use were also linked to changes in other health practices such as increases in safer-sex practices or reductions in violent behaviors. For example, it was not uncommon for men to articulate that their improvements in condom use or reductions in the number of sexual partners were linked to reductions in the volume of alcohol they imbibed:

> One Man Can changed me for the better. . . . [I]t has made me a better man because now if I feel I have had enough to drink I go home, as opposed to the earlier habits of going to see girlfriends. That was risky because I was putting myself at risk of unprotected sex and HIV. I have also reduced on the amount of alcohol that I consume. (Eastern Cape, age 19, single)

It was also not uncommon for men to describe that their own reductions in alcohol use helped to facilitate reduced violence against women and other household members:

> Before I joined One Man Can, I could drink for three consecutive days. I was also violent in my drunken states and I would sometimes physically assault my girlfriend and would also treat other household members roughly. Since I became involved with One Man Can, I am able to go for a month without having a single drink of alcohol. Now I respect my girlfriend and if I have to go and see her, I make sure that I am in a sober state and that I also respect her wishes if she wants us to use protection during sex. (Eastern Cape, age 44, married)

Another man reported,

> I was one of the people who used to practice domestic violence before I
> was part of One Man Can. In my digital story, I did not conceal the fact
> that I was once sentenced to a five month imprisonment for domestic
> violence. I was drunk at the time. However since becoming part of One
> Man Can I changed a lot. In the community when domestic violence
> happens, I am able to intervene in domestic violence situations. (Eastern
> Cape, age 33, single)

One-quarter of the men in our sample were members of a "community-
action team" (CAT) who took the gender and health issues that were most
important to their local communities and worked on these collectively.
One of the themes from a CAT that men described focused on alcohol use
in the community, with men seeking to press beyond an individual focus
and ensure that the availability of alcohol was curtailed at a broader level.
Thus, several men not only stated that they individually cut down on alcohol consumption but also explained the way that they formed a team that
negotiated with tavern owners in their respective communities to close
bars (*shebeens*) early. These men believed that because so much unsafe
sex and violence ensued at taverns (or after their close), cutting back on
the hours of the tavern could cut back on the volume of alcohol that is
consumed, and this could have a major impact on violence and unsafe sex.
Tavern owners complied in these instances, at least in the short term, but
this was extremely challenging given a fear of lost profits—and was probably only possible because of the number of community members who
fought for this change. However, we did not carry out long-term follow-
up interviews to see if these changes in social practice at the community
level were maintained over time. It is interesting, however, to see how the
workshops sparked, supported, and facilitated community-level mobilization and how masculinities were then reshaped in terms of collective and
institutional practices and not just at the individual level.

In addition to men articulating that shifts in alcohol use led to
changes in unsafe-sex and violence-related behaviors, men also articulated how reductions in drinking facilitated a more positive relationship
with their children and partners. For example, it was not uncommon for
them to describe changes such as the following:

One Man Can helped me in that regard because I was a person that used to like fun and drinking alcohol. I was always out there with the boys drinking. I didn't have time for my girlfriend and my daughter. She would come with my daughter to the tavern and beg me to at least give them attention. Sometimes she would go to my place and find me absent and she would sleep and wait for me. On my arrival, I would get into arguments with her. However after that workshop, I got to understand the importance of care and it has helped me. I am also enjoying it as well. One Man Can changed the way I live my life and the decisions that I make as a man. (Eastern Cape, age 23, single)

These kinds of changes help us to understand that men shifted their own social opportunity structures, challenging the kinds of norms and practices that men engaged in within particular spaces (bars, homosocial spaces with other men, etc.).

Discussions of violence were, of course, not always linked to alcohol use. Many men in our sample underscored that OMC specifically shifted their understanding of the link among male-dominated decision making, violent behavior, and masculine respect (that violence is needed to maintain masculine respect). This came through very clearly in narratives that were focused on violence against not only women but also children and other men. Men described reductions in the use of violence against women and how they garnered newfound understanding that heated emotions, anger, or violations of gender-norm expectations were not a license to enact violence:

One Man Can changed me in a way because it changed my own relationship. If my girlfriend is angry with me and even if she is the one that is wrong, I calm down and talk to her without fighting. I respect her and I know that I should not beat her up. She even told me that things have changed in the way I act in our relationship and she is happy about that. (Eastern Cape, age 34, single)

Men in the workshops were challenged to think about why, when they are angry at their boss at work, they don't hit their boss, but when they are angry at their female partners or men outside of the workplace, they consider violence as a solution (Sonke Gender Justice 2012). Indeed, workshop facilitators encouraged men to think critically about the links between violence and notions of masculine respect. The same was true with regard to men's relationships with their children. Several men in our sample explained that they shifted from equating masculinity, toughness, and corporal punishment to an ethic of care:

> One Man Can changed a lot of things in me. I used to be the kind of person who was feared in the village by young people because of my tough reputation. I was the kind of man whom, when a child cries would be told "I will call him" and the child would go quiet. The training I got from One Man Can changed me in a way that I was taught not to intimidate children but to be more caring to them. (Eastern Cape, age 41, single)

Many fathers in the Eastern Cape in particular reported to us that they used fewer corporal discipline strategies with their children because of their participation in OMC. OMC allowed for a better understanding of the effects of harsh discipline on children and encouraged more talking with and listening to children. For example, one father who had been raised with harsh physical abuse and imposed that on his children reflected on this change: "I was previously a very strict man and a disciplinarian. In being strict, I have to admit that I was also rough, but those young men at Sonke taught us different ways of disciplining children" (Eastern Cape, age 54, married).

Unhinging masculinity from notions of being feared and respected was one of the main goals of one of the One Man Can workshops, titled "A Live Fool or a Dead Hero?" In it, men were challenged to decouple masculinity from a willingness to die in the name of not backing down during instances of male-on-male violence. Indeed, several men narrated that participation in OMC helped them to reduce violent behavior with other men:

> I am a person who used to like fighting. Men in rural areas view fighting as a measure of manhood and competition. What we do not realize is the risk associated with fighting because many a time people get seriously injured or even die during these fights. That One Man Can program made me realize that there are other alternatives to fighting and thus if a person does something wrong and apologizes, I do accept the apology. (Eastern Cape, age 31, married)

The same tactics were used in sessions designed to reduce violence against women and encourage more equitable relationships. Instead of seeking to constitute masculinity through fear, distance, dominance, and respect defended with violence, men were challenged to think about the benefits of a relationship that did not involve physical abuse—both for themselves and for their partners:

> I used to consume a lot of alcohol and did not care about other people. Being a part of One Man Can was eye opening because it opened my eyes to the negative effects of my previous behavior. Because of One Man Can, I think relationships are supposed to make people happy and love each other, rather than make them unhappy and be abused. One Man Can also encouraged people in a relationship to communicate as it can help to avoid physical fights. (Eastern Cape, age 33, single)

It is critical to recall once more that masculinity in One Man Can was viewed not only as an individual-level set of norms and practices but also as a community-level set of social practices that is embedded in a vibrant civil society. Here, men in One Man Can described how they saw themselves as playing an active role in intervening in violence against women and children not only at the individual level but also at the community level. Several men in our study reported that they made attempts to intervene in these injustices when witnessed. For example, several men reported themes such as the following:

> We are lucky in this community because we are united and thus information spreads faster. The men who attended One Man Can training sessions made an awareness campaign on domestic violence and on the importance of not beating up one's partner. People were encouraged to fix things by communicating because the stick does not build a home. I can safely say that gender violence is not as common now but if it does happen, the community acts. For us, screaming means someone is in danger and thus we have to act. If we wake up and find that a man is beating up his wife, we become angry because he is not supposed to do that. As a community we are fighting against violence. We men who were part of One Man Can were taught how to handle such situations. We do not care who is fighting, we intervene. (Eastern Cape, age 27, single)

Several men in our Limpopo sample also reported that because of their participation in OMC, after the OMC workshops, men began door-to-door campaigns to stop violence against women and children in their respective communities. In the door-to-door campaigns, a group of men visited households in their communities and encouraged men to emotionally support women and daughters after rape and also encouraged women to report rape cases to the police. Despite research in South Africa that finds that women are very unlikely to report rape and that the police are often unresponsive to reports (Kapp 2006), men in our sample perceived that this door-to-door campaign helped to reduce violence against women and children in their respective communities.

Simultaneously, several men in our sample reported that they were, at times, afraid to stop male-female violence when they witnessed it publicly because they feared that the violent male partner would assume that they themselves were having an affair with the woman. These men therefore feared that the violence would transfer to them in their effort to stop it and that their lives might be put at risk in the process. Thus, men in our sample were grateful to have learned that they could take a more active role in stopping violence but also expressed that they were afraid to intervene on some male-female and male-on-male violence for fear of risk to themselves. Nonetheless, several men in our sample did describe scenarios in which they intervened to stop acts of violence, whether these incidents sought to harm women or men. In the words of one man,

> Young men play with fighting. But one day, there were these two young men who were pushed to fight. Usually a fight will take 10 to 15 minutes maximum. But that one became too long, something like 30 to 40 minutes. These young men were strongly punching each other to a river of blood. I then went in to stop the boys. To me I think I saved souls if not a soul. These boys were going to kill each other. (Limpopo, age 27, unmarried)

Men described not only reductions in violence against women and men and in alcohol use but also reductions in the number of sexual partners and increased condom use. Here, similarly to the way men narrated changes in relationship power where they increasingly valued women's

contributions to household decisions, OMC was described as influencing men's ability to hear and respond positively to women's requests for
condom use: "As a result of One Man Can, I realized the importance
of using a condom and my girlfriend was happy about it because she
had been encouraging me all along to use a condom. In One Man Can,
we were taught about the risks one exposes himself to if they do not
use condoms" (Eastern Cape, age 19, single). Other men talked about
how prior to OMC, they did not see the importance of using a condom during sex either because this would interrupt pleasure and make
them feel like less of a man or because men perceived that HIV and
AIDS did not originate in South Africa. The OMC program helped
men to challenge common connections that men made between sexual
protection and masculinity (i.e., that you're not a real man if you use
a condom) and also challenged ideas that men had about HIV being
caused by "foreigners":

> Things have changed for me my brother. First, I was not using a condom
> because things like HIV and AIDS we used to see them on television
> short stories thinking that it is not here in South Africa. . . . [W]e thought
> it was being brought by foreigners. Now I find that each and everyone you
> meet, you must condomize. (Eastern Cape, age 25, single)

Several men were very clear that the workshops helped them to reconfigure definitions of masculinity that equated manhood with multiple
partners:

> To be honest with you, I was a person who did not admire a man who
> was loyal to one girlfriend. I viewed such men as weak, desperate, and
> being *isishumane* [a man who cannot get a girlfriend]. My view was that
> to be respected by other men one should be involved with at least three
> women. However since I started OMC, I took the decision to have one
> partner and be loyal to that partner. (Eastern Cape, age 41, married)

What is so interesting about the narrative above is that it underscores
the importance of gender as not only vertically defined in relation to
women but also horizontally defined in relation to other men—and
shows that vertical definitions of masculinity influence health. That is,

prior to OMC, it was not simply that having many female sexual partners constituted masculinity for any given individual man but that it
does so collectively in the eyes of other men. Thus, men "do masculinity" through multiple partners not only to bolster their own individual
status or self-esteem but also to bolster masculinity as a collective practice that is witnessed by women and other men.

Many men in our sample also explained that OMC helped them to
talk with their partners about safe sex and also opened them up to the
possibility of HIV testing. And, one-third of our sample of men reported
that because of participation in One Man Can, they received an HIV
test. Men explained to us that

> One Man Can helped me and my partner to open up and share about
> important things like sexually transmitted diseases and condom usage.
> My partner and I have agreed to use condoms whenever we have sex. Let
> me be honest with you: I always tell my partner that whenever she gets
> tempted somewhere out there she must use a condom. You never know
> what will happen out there. We are human. My wife and I talk about it of-
> ten. Last Wednesday, we talked about sexually transmitted diseases. And
> above all, my partner and I are going to have HIV tests together. These are
> One Man Can achievements for me. (Limpopo, age 32, married)

Thus far in this chapter, I have detailed several historical and contextual
aspects of South African society and have provided some information
on race, class, gender, and sexuality relations in contemporary South
Africa. I have provided coverage that described the HIV/AIDS epidemic
in South Africa. I have examined the perceived impact that this particular gender-transformative health program had on men's views of gender
relations, masculinities, and their alcohol, HIV-related, and violence
practices. This study overall attempted to answer the question of how
men respond to being asked to change in the direction of more gender equality in the name of improved health. One Man Can, a women's
rights–based and masculinities-focused HIV- and violence-prevention
program, appeared to positively shift many men's ideologies about gender relations, masculinities, and perceptions of women's rights. These
changes were not limited to beliefs but were also infused into emergent practices. Men described shifts in the direction of more gender

equality within relationships with women and children. In addition, men's changes in gender ideologies and notions of manhood appeared to be intertwined with a number of improved health practices, including reduced alcohol intake, increased condom use, reduction in the number of partners, increased HIV testing, and decreased violence against women, men, and children. Our results overall do seem consistent with the results of those who argue that gender-transformative programming can play an important role in engaging men as active agents who can and do play a meaningful role in reshaping equality and health for both women and men (Barker, Ricardo, & Nascimento 2007; Dworkin et al. 2011, 2012; Dworkin, Hatcher et al. 2013; Dworkin, Treves-Kagan, & Lippman 2013; Peacock, Khumalo, & McNab 2006; Peacock 2013; Pulerwitz & Barker 2008; van den Berg et al. 2013). To this, I would add that such programs appear promising for improving men's relationship with children and reducing abuse with children as well.

Simultaneously, men articulated a number of challenges to gender-transformative programming that should be considered. First, a few men articulated that they are upset about the way that the program is designed to examine gender relations but is only carried out with men as central to it (and not women). Here, recall my previous points in chapter 3 that even though gender is relational, it is common for programming to be implemented as either male-only or female-only programming. A few men saw this as particularly problematic in the case of OMC. In the words of one man, "The one thing men ask about most is why OMC is focused on men only. Men think that this is a form of making men culprits and they have shown their displeasure at the viewpoint that men are the [perpetrators] of abuse and violence" (Eastern Cape, age 35, single). This is an important point, because thousands of evaluated health-promotion and health-serviced-based programs have "included men and boys as target populations but have not fully considered how gender norms affect the health-related behaviors, attitudes, and vulnerabilities of men and women" (Barker et al. 2010, 540). Indeed, even within gender-transformative programs that do focus on how gender norms affect men, researchers inadvertently risk essentializing "problematic" aspects of masculinities, reducing these to individual traits and potentially leaving men feeling blamed for HIV and violence in their communities. This can occur particularly when programs do not centrally recognize the structural, institutional, cultural, or interpersonal aspects of their lives that shape their notions of what it means to be a man.

To be clear, Sonke's programming explicitly attempted to press beyond notions of masculinity as static, singular, individualized, and/or decontextualized, and it did so in a few critical ways that are worth highlighting. First, as I've already emphasized, OMC attempted to focus on the way gender inequality shapes women's and men's health while also focusing on the costs to men and women of adhering to narrow and constraining definitions of masculinity. In this way, men were positioned not only as "beneficiaries" in the gender order (a point made in chapter 2) but also as a group that can also be harmed in gender relations. Because of the ways in which men do adhere to narrow definitions of masculinity (in the name of being "real men"), it was the case that men in Sonke's workshops talked with one another about how they recognized that they can become injured or die in fights with other men, how they can lose out on women's input into households, relationships, and communities, and how they can miss out on experiences of love, closeness, and connectedness with their partners and children. And because OMC challenged strict adherence to ideas about "being a real man," men challenged some of their own social practices, which included self-constituting as masculine through their health practices by drinking too much, enacting violence, or engaging in high-risk sex. Thus, men's participation in a shift towards gender equality became understood in terms of its benefits not only for women but also for men—and not only for themselves but also for their families and communities.

Second, OMC recognized not only that gender relations shape masculinities but also that the history of race relations in South African society shapes the specificities of masculinities. In the conversations about gender relations in Sonke's One Man Can workshops, men were connecting experiences of racial inequality with experiences of gender inequality, and thus, men had emergent realizations and recognition of how injustice works to situate people as inferior (no matter what the social location). For example, we saw that men in this sample talked about how oppressive race relations in the country had been reconfigured and about how all people deserve equal rights. We saw in this chapter that some men stated that they "know what it is like" to be treated in as inferior on the basis of race and that gender inequality therefore also should have no place in South African society. This emphasis and the long history of racial inequality in South Africa helped some men to see racial and gender injustice as a societal-level phenomenon that is constituted by people in power and through social relations that can be dismantled or fought. A critical point here is that gender-transformative programming has not taken up the primacy of race and class relations in order to reduce HIV risks or improve HIV care, treatment, or testing outcomes. However, these men's narratives point us to how intersectional logic might be usefully integrated into such programs in the future to engage men and to help shift them in the direction of gender equality (without making them feel blamed for gender inequality).

Third, OMC pressed against fixed notions of men as recalcitrant to change or as an individual-level problem by engaging men as positive agents of change not only in their relationships but also in terms of their emerging social practices in local communities. Several men took what they had learned with other men in the workshops and participated as active agents of change beyond the small-group level by participating in community action teams. Here, men engaged tavern owners to reduce violence and HIV risks at the community level or started a door-to-door campaign to stop violence against women and children. Thus, rather than view OMC as offering a one-size-fits-all, "universal" set of strategies for social change that can improve health, the program facilitators asked community members to prioritize the gender-equality and health-related practices that were relevant to women and men in particular locales given men's embeddedness in local social relations.

But some men still felt blamed for violence in their communities and for high HIV rates. Even if Sonke's programming succeeded at shifting away from classic one-shot public-health workshops to stimulate broader community mobilization, it is critical to recall that communities are still contextualized in stratified social relations where the norms and practices of hegemonic masculinity, while not overdetermined, may still be more highly valued than those of subordinated masculinities. Hence, public- and global-health scholars might benefit from social science research such as this (and Wyrod 2008; Wyrod 2016), which underscores that one can expect contestation, debate, and resistance on the ground about masculinities and women's rights, given long histories of social relations, rather than any kind of sudden, linear, or overnight change.

Along these lines, a few men in our study did state in interviews that they were honestly confused by the materials that were shared and reflected upon in One Man Can workshops. This is the case because once men internalized the main messages of the workshops and shifted in the direction of more gender equality in their relationships and communities, there were other men in their communities who did not attend OMC and belittled or humiliated the participants. In the words of one man, "It confuses me completely, especially in my community. I end up convincing myself that I am wrong with my new, right understanding that men are partners to women and not rulers of women" (Limpopo, age 29, single). Thus, again, understanding gender relations and the way they influence health involves not only a relational understanding of women and men but also an understanding of the construction of gender among men (Connell 1987, 1995a; Messner 1997, 2002). It is therefore critical to consider the way gender equality is not just about the way men treat women but also about how some men enact social control over other men concerning the boundaries of masculinities. Indeed, a few men described feeling policed and even humiliated by other men when they tried out new, more equitable practices in their relationships and communities:

> What happened is that after the One Man Can workshop, I met other guys in the village and had conversations with other men about what we had been taught at the One Man Can workshop. I told them that even men can wash the baby nappies and take care of children. I cannot describe the reaction but all I can say is that they were shocked. After that, they then told me that I am a sissy boy, a softie, and some even suggested that I am gay. They looked down upon me and that really made me feel humiliated and less of a man. (Eastern Cape, age 27, single)

Previous social science scholarship has highlighted the way in which men police the norms and practices of masculinity through teasing, humiliation, social control, and even violence against other men (Dorais & Lajeunesse 2004; Pascoe 2011). Scholars working to advance gender equality in the name of health have argued that positive social valuations of "changed men" (who are more gender equitable) can be built through using a strategy of putting forward "positive role models"

(Barker 2008; Barker, Ricardo, & Nascimento 2007; Peacock & Levack 2004; Pulerwitz, Michaelis, et al. 2010). My own systematic review of gender-transformative interventions with colleagues (Dworkin, Treves-Kagan, & Lippman 2013) and the work in this chapter also suggest that it can be important to consider shifting beyond single-shot public-health workshop models to include community-level mobilization as a promising route through which changes in normative conceptions of masculinities (or other valued social ideals) can occur. This makes it more likely that individual men won't face humiliation or more severe consequences for enacting shifts in the direction of more gender equality. While Sonke's One Man Can program does incorporate a community-mobilization process through community action teams (CATs), as I mentioned, we did not study this element of the program beyond post-program individual interviews or over time. We did not deeply evaluate the community-mobilization elements that occurred among men who participated in CATs as they interacted with their communities and families. Thus, we understand less than we'd like to about how men were received by their partners at home or by other women and men in the community at large. This knowledge would be critical to garnering a more full understanding of masculinity as a collective and institutional set of practices.

At the same time that a few men described how their peers were resistant to their changed beliefs and social practices, some men also reported that they stood up to men who attempted to chastise or humiliate them. This theme is reflected in the following statement:

> I am very satisfied and I am happy when I am with my family because I don't go out a lot. Other men sometimes laugh at me and say that I like being at home like I am a kitchen utensil. So I have changed a lot, because I am this man who is around his wife, and other men do complain that I am spending most of my time with my wife. But I continue practicing that and I will not change. (Eastern Cape, age 54, married)

It is unclear whether the ability to stand up to this type of social pressure was age dependent, but it may be the case that younger men reported less resilience to standing up to normative conceptions of masculinity compared to older men. Indeed, perhaps readers have noticed that many narratives of younger men are not in our descriptions of "change" because younger men (aged eighteen to twenty-four) did not narrate as many changes in masculinity and health practices.

Also consistent with concepts of intersectionality was that younger men stated to us in the interviews that they wanted workshops to be for young men only because of age hierarchies in South Africa, where respect for older men is highly valued and contestation exists across generations. These hierarchies may have led young men to speak much less in a group setting that included older men. When I presented research to Sonke colleagues in Cape Town, South Africa, showing that young men were less likely to make health-behavior changes than older men, they stated that in the future they would consider structuring the group workshops on the basis of age. Indeed, this recommendation is consistent with research that calls for HIV prevention among young men in South Africa to focus on "shifting the norms of masculinity in which male partner violence is rooted" (Jewkes et al. 2011).

In addition to the above challenges that are associated with carrying out gender-transformative health programming, there are also specific methodological limitations to this work that deserve some attention. One set of limitations in the current work is that for several reasons we cannot determine definitively whether this program resulted in improved gender equality or improved health outcomes. Participants may certainly be subject to response bias, attempting to put their best foot forward when asked questions. To minimize this bias, interviewers were hired who were external to Sonke but lived in the local area and were not perceived as part of the original programming. In addition, our participants were not randomized into this program, and there was no control group, so selection bias is operating (men who self-select into this study may be more gender equitable to begin with than men who don't). And, this is a postintervention study, so there were no pre-/post-test results on equality or health outcomes that would more definitively help us to understand ideas at "baseline" and "follow-up" about emergent social practices and change. I provided some results from a similar sample of men in order to attempt to get at "baseline"-level data, but this was an imperfect method of comparison to use across these two samples. And, while we qualitatively explored topics related to gender relations, women's rights, gendered power, masculinities, safe sex, violence, and alcohol, we did not use quantitative measures to characterize health outcomes or gender equality. Lastly, we carried out one interview at one time point (postintervention), and we do not have a longitudinally designed study. As was discussed, we did not use ethnography to examine how men were received in their relationships and communities when they arrived to try out new social practices consistent with gender equality and health. At the same time that we recognize these weaknesses, the current study was critically important to understanding men's subjectivities concerning how they respond within gender-transformative programming to being asked to reshape norms of masculinities and to embrace gender equality in the name of fighting violence against women and men and reducing HIV risks in South Africa.

Finally, despite all of the conceptual understanding that OMC developers and implementers have about masculinity as a collective practice and as contextually and historically shaped, a few men who participated in the program still felt that men were being viewed negatively and singled out as "bad" individual men. Recall how, earlier in this chapter, I quoted men who referred to the impact of OMC as helping them to realize the "negative effects of my previous behavior." Recall also that there were many men whose statements were consistent with the message that OMC "has made me a better man," implying that they were now "different" or somehow "improved" men because they reported leaving taverns early, drinking less, going home earlier at night, reducing violence against women, children, family members, and other men, and increasing condom use with their sexual partners or cutting back on the number of partners. These types of narratives indicate a potential move away from a contextualized understanding of masculinities as racialized, classed, and structurally, historically, and culturally shaped (Hunter 2005, 2007; Morrell 1998, 2002; Richter & Morrell 2006) and towards a view of masculinity as a problem to be solved by making men into what might be called "responsibilized citizens" who take the initiative to change their own health through a variety of lifestyle changes (Barry, Osborne, & Rose 1996; Colvin, Robins, & Leavens 2010; Robins 2008a). While some degree of agency is certainly implied in this concept, at first glance, it may also seem to have something in common with analyses that critique public health as a moralizing or confessional set of disciplinary health practices (Campos et al. 2006; Crawford 1980; Foucault 1980; Petersen & Lupton 1996).

Thus, despite the rights-based and social-justice emphasis in which gendered power, women's empowerment, and the costs of masculinities to women and men were frequently emphasized in OMC, these narratives reveal some of the ways in which the content or the interpretation of content reflected public health language of "behavior" and individual blame. These notions have both long been critiqued by social scientists, anthropologists, and some public-health and global-health scholars alike. What men are telling us in this research, then, is that some of them may feel individually and collectively responsible for changing their own masculinity—and the manhood of others—rather than being offered the recognition (or a different intervention that would intervene on the fact) that there are larger and complex social and institutional forces that shape masculinities—and will also reshape them. Ultimately, then, OMC viewed men positively as having critical assets to draw upon, and, of importance, recognized them as agentic, rallying for gendered social justice and transformative social and health-related change. Simultaneously, perhaps some men were telling us that, in a program called "One Man Can," they perceived that they were being asked to shoulder the required shifts in citizenship that are needed to build equality and health in their local communities.

While I have attempted to make a nuanced case for the importance and powerful impact of gender-transformative health programming, I hope that readers will now join me in thinking much more critically about what it means when NGO and global-health programming asks race- and class-marginalized men themselves to carry the weight of shifting violence, HIV, and gender-equality outcomes in South African society and beyond. Does this mean that men were disciplined objects in a neoliberal environment, internalizing health as the highest value (Crawford 1980; Dworkin & Wachs 2009; Lupton 1995), directing their energies to self-regulation and self-improvement? Were they asked to do so even as they were suffering from unemployment, poverty, and other cumulative histories that have resulted partly from a "ruthless" and "racist minority" (Thompson 2000) and retractions in state spending that arrived with globalization processes (Bond 2000)? Does this mean that the men in this gender-transformative program were subject to the disciplinary gaze of the state enjoining them to take responsibility for their own health, coupled with rights-based discourses that may have been imposed from the West? Or does this mean something else entirely about HIV and violence prevention in South Africa and beyond? That is the focus of the next and final chapter. This last chapter will be the first piece of published work that moves beyond success stories in gender-transformative programs with men. I do so not because I don't believe in the very real positive impact of gender-transformative programs that I've detailed in this chapter and that is revealed in other published work. I do so in order to critically reflect on the promises and limitations of this kind of programming—to think about what success really means in gender-transformative programs—and to consider where the interdisciplinary field of HIV prevention with heterosexually active men might go next.

5

"Being a Better Man"

Masculinities and Gender Transformation in HIV- and Violence-
Prevention Programs

In this book, I have attempted to carry out several conceptual and empirical tasks. Throughout the past four chapters, I have drawn upon sociological perspectives that are central to gender and feminist studies, and have offered a critical perspective on public- and global-health literatures and programs. I have carried out a rigorous assessment of the HIV-prevention literature on men, and I have attempted to critically assess how heterosexually active men are often omitted from the science base concerning behavioral HIV-prevention interventions both domestically and globally. Indeed, in the United States, we are in the fourth decade of the epidemic, and scholars have made it very clear that the intersecting dynamics of gender, race, class, and sexuality produce "heterosexual sex" as the largest category of transmission in the world. But, heterosexually active men are not often understood within the HIV/AIDS-prevention science base as having gender or being affected by masculinity and gender relations (for a few exceptions see the systematic review by Dworkin, Treves-Kagan, & Lippman 2013). In the global realm, where masculinities-based work with heterosexually active men is more common than it is in the United States, interventions are rarely designed to attend to structurally produced race, class, and gender inequalities that men experience and that shape their vulnerabilities to HIV.

In order to assess this situation and consider why this might be occurring, I drew upon my own work and a collaboration with colleagues at Columbia University in which we critically assessed the conceptual underpinnings of a "vulnerability paradigm" that is often deployed in prevention interventions with heterosexually active women and men (Dworkin 2005; Higgins, Hoffman, & Dworkin 2010). I examined the history and trajectory of the vulnerability paradigm that challenged the assertion that heterosexually active men are not "vulnerable" to HIV risks. I have argued throughout this work that domestic HIV-prevention interventions with heterosexually active men have quite a ways to travel in order to consistently recognize masculinities and gender relations as shaping men's HIV risks and violence practices. I've also argued that both domestically and globally, frameworks that take the intersectional nature of privilege and oppression into account would go a long way in pressing beyond gender as the privileged axis of intervention. I then described common responses to the HIV pandemic in terms of prevention programs and fleshed out the promises and limitations of women-only (women's empowerment) and men-only (men as partners—and gender-transformative) programs that are responsive to the interrelated HIV and violence epidemics. I made suggestions concerning how the benefits of each of these lines of work could simultaneously be drawn upon to synergistically improve HIV-prevention interventions. Out of this analysis, I argued that gender should be increasingly seen as relational and that interventions might fruitfully consider carrying out more interventions with women and men side by side in future programming.

In addition, throughout *Men at Risk*, I've attempted to draw on social science insights into masculinities, gender relations, and sexuality to underscore that research generally draws upon, or even uncritically deploys, a sex-gender-sexuality triad in HIV prevention. This triad generally assumes that men are powerful and are privileged in the gender order and views men as having an uncontrollable and natural essence to their sexuality that must be brought under control by their having fewer partners, sticking to one partner, or using condoms. Gender-transformative work presses beyond these limitations by recognizing that masculinity is not a fixed essence but is socially shaped and constrained, and views men as agents of positive change in their intimate relationships, families, and communities.

Within *Men at Risk*, I've also been clear that there are disjunctures between sexual acts and sexual identities and that little HIV-prevention work that is directed at heterosexually identified men domestically and globally in the science base even acknowledges that men may have not only female partners but also male partners. In chapter 2, I examined research that shows that many men might identify as heterosexually active but have both male and female partners. And the same is true in

South Africa and elsewhere. Research in South Africa by Kristin Dunkle and colleagues shows that in a population-based household survey, one in twenty men admit to having a consensual sexual relationship with a man and nearly all of these men have a female partner. In that study, one in ten men had experienced sexual assault by another man, and men who had had any type of sex with men were significantly more likely to be HIV positive (Dunkle et al. 2011). Thus, when thinking about gender-transformative programming with heterosexually active men, both domestic and global, we do not yet know if the conceptual basis for "transforming gender" is helpful only to men's intimate relations with women, or if this would be useful with men's male partners as well. We don't know if gender-transformative work reduces risk with female partners but not male partners, although such work could certainly be modified to more appropriately focus on both.

While the promises and limitations of gender-transformative interventions have been laid out in depth, particularly in chapter 4, I also underscored in chapter 1 and chapter 4 that the limitations of gender-neutral HIV-prevention programming are vast and that gender-transformative work radically reduces these limitations. Because of the volume of literature that makes clear that social constructions of masculinity do impact men's and women's health, particularly in terms of violence and HIV outcomes, it is critical to not assume that gender-neutral HIV-prevention strategies adequately take men's (and by extension, women's) HIV and violence risks into account. Indeed, gender-sensitive and gender-transformative interventions have been shown to be driven by concepts focused on masculinities and gender relations that show much promise and success in increasing protective sexual behaviors, preventing partner violence, changing negative attitudes towards women, shifting notions of masculinity, and reducing STI/HIV risks (Dworkin, Treves-Kagan, & Lippman 2013).

Some gender-transformative HIV- and violence-prevention interventions are particularly intriguing and important both conceptually and in their implementation, practice, and impacts, including the One Man Can program based at Sonke Gender Justice in South Africa. Such programs do not simply argue that men are harmed in the gender order (i.e., "costs of masculinity") but also pay nuanced attention to the fact that many men enjoy social, cultural, and normative privileges that negatively shape both women's and men's health. Because of this recognition, some gender-transformative HIV- and violence-prevention programs such as One Man Can work to shift norms of masculinities, minimize inequalities between women and men, and challenge men to move in the direction of more gender equality in the name of social justice and improved health. This and other on-the-ground approaches in South Africa and elsewhere are increasingly embedded "in a growing body of literature on African masculinities that challenges essentialist and ahistorical conceptions of a singular African masculinity and sexuality" (Colvin, Robins, & Leavens 2010, 1186). One Man Can is one such program.

One Man Can was influenced by numerous women's rights organizations and feminist colleagues and is designed by women and men working together on the ground in South Africa. Such colleagues are acutely aware of the intersecting history of colonialism, apartheid, migratory movements, poverty, and gender inequality, drawing upon the ways in which men's notions of masculinity and gender equality are linked to health. The program as it is implemented also facilitates important conversations among men that emerge organically and that link racial inequality and gender inequality when attempting to understand the reason for violence outcomes and HIV prevention, treatment, and care outcomes. As was seen in chapter 4, men related deeply to the topic of racial inequality given the history of race relations and their life experiences, and they were engaged by ideas that challenged their understanding of women's rights, gender equality, and masculinities. Transforming gender relations in the workshops and beyond ultimately seemed to have numerous positive impacts on norms of masculinity and positive health effects, including reduced alcohol use, violence, and HIV-risk and HIV-testing behaviors.

While chapter 4 revealed many areas of individual and community-level success, there are still some important questions about gender-transformative work that deserve attention. These comments are meant to assist researchers, practitioners, and others in the field in thinking about the future of gender-transformative programming. For example, within gender-transformative programs, what should the balance be between workshop material that focuses on the "costs of masculinities" to women and men and program content that focuses on how men enjoy "social and institutional privileges" as a group (Messner 1997)? Both of these areas of content are known to shape health outcomes for women and men. What should the balance be between these materials and materials that emphasize the "differences and inequalities among men," which point to the need to understand the concept of intersectionality and point to the question of why some men are so much more impacted by HIV and violence than other men? All of these conceptual arms that help to fully explain masculinities as a set of ideologies and practices—costs of masculinity, social and institutional privileges, and differences and inequalities among men (Messner 1997)—form the basis for a much richer understanding of masculinities than does emphasis on any one or two of these arms. We can and should be more reflective in HIV-prevention, -treatment, and -care programs concerning the emphasis that is given to the substantive content in each of these areas and how to tailor this content for different groups of men.

While Sonke's One Man Can certainly made attempts to focus explicitly on two of the above arms (social and institutional privileges and the costs of masculinity) and appears to have successfully engaged many men in terms of social justice, gender equality, and health, questions do remain about how much one arm is emphasized over the other in this and other gender-transformative programs. We don't know what the impacts would be on gender equality and health if certain arms of this theoretical triad were emphasized more than others. In our empirical study, it was not always easy to garner how men articulated their experiences as linked or unlinked across these arms, and questions in the interview guide were not fully directed at these interrelationships. Future research could bolster an understanding of how gender-transformative programming is shaped by these three arms of thinking and could examine the impact that different emphases have in shaping gender equality and health outcomes in various regions.

These results make it clear that it is critical for global health and public health researchers to collaborate with social science researchers in designing and assessing HIV-prevention science. Currently, it is common in gender-transformative programs to examine short-term improvements in the gender-equitable man scale or gender-norms scale and to examine whether these improvements explain reductions in violence or HIV risk. However, as has been argued in chapter 4, it is also important to examine how women and men struggle with and deploy, over time, new notions of femininities and masculinities in their house-holds, relationships, and communities. These enactments arise out of shifting gender relations and participation in health programs that are centered on women's empowerment and/or gender-transformative pro-gramming. This is particularly important given the work in chapters 2 and 4, which underscores the ways in which masculinities are racialized.

In addition, the field has very little knowledge about how women or men are received by their peers, parents, families, and community mem-bers when they make changes in their lives that shift in the direction of more gender equality. It may be the case that men are welcomed when they shift towards more gender-equitable beliefs and practices. But they may also be humiliated, be belittled, or have their behaviors policed by others around them. And, it may be the case that women who partici-pate in women's empowerment programming or gender-transformative programming are welcomed by their peers, male partners, and com-munity members when they enact agency, reject gender-inequitable at-titudes or practices, and enjoy more structural or interpersonal power. But they may also experience masculinism and/or backlash in limited or extreme forms from family members, friends, partners, or others. Currently, we just do not know enough about the processual nature of gender relations and the contested nature of gender equality at the close of health-related programs in areas where programs are implemented. This would be particularly important to flesh out within future struc-tural interventions that are directed at men.

In addition, HIV research does not often enough study ongoing gender-transformative work at the community level nor investigate how community-mobilization processes form, are stabilized, are fraught, or are impossible to maintain—because such analysis is a long-term, expensive, and complex endeavor. Studies are now attempting to measure "com-munity mobilization" quantitatively and to see if these processes matter for reduced violence and HIV risks. This is important and newly funded work, and results will be published by a team including Sonke, Sheri Lippman at UCSF, and Audrey Pettifor at UNC–Chapel Hill. Indeed, it is critical to keep in mind that health-related programs with or without community-mobilization elements are embedded in a socioeconomic, so-ciopolitical, and cultural context whereby the intersections of race, class, gender, and sexuality relations were changing prior to interventions and will shift afterward as well. Thus, rich ethnographic and social science work that sheds light on the contexts in which health programs are being implemented, the unique forms and content of community mobilization, and its reach and impact on health needs to be examined.

The influence of social science work on public and global health work in HIV prevention has been critical in pressing researchers to be a bit more mindful about essentializing men as individually uncaring, irresponsible, violent, untrustworthy, and disinterested in women's rights, or as being unworthy of attempts to change them. As I described in chapter 1, Barker and colleagues (2010) underscore that health programs often view "men mainly as oppressors—self-centered, disinterested, or violent—instead of as complex subjects whose behaviors are influenced by gender and sexual norms" (540). Indeed, as I have shown, even within gender-transformative programs where men are not directly viewed in these ways (and are seen as being shaped by gender, race, class, and sexual norms), researchers risk essentializing "problematic" aspects of masculinities, reducing these to individual traits, leaving men feeling blamed for HIV and violence in their communities. Thus, despite the fact that gender-transformative work can be grounded in complex literature on masculinities in a given region, it can have the inadvertent consequences of coming across to men as a moral call for men to unlearn certain forms of male socialization that are being inadvertently blamed for inequality and health problems.

It is critical to think about whether researchers and practitioners of gender-transformative programs are inadvertently individualizing (or collectivizing) masculinity as a problem that needs to be fixed as opposed to a collective set of practices that require institutional, cultural, community-level, legal, occupational, and policy support. Similar questions have been posed when researchers critically assess the value of turning to women and asking them to individually change in the name of improved health. For example, similar questions have been previously raised about the transition from gender-neutral to more gender-sensitive and gender-empowering work with women (Exner et al. 2003). Another example is the way global feminists questioned the use of microfinance as a solution to women's disempowerment and the negative health outcomes that result from poverty because these problems are partly driven by neoliberal globalization, privatization, macro-level trade policies, and power relations between the Global North and the Global South. Scholars have argued that the solution to enormous social processes associated with poverty and development should not rest on the shoulders of individual women alone in the context of these broader and massive shifts (Karim 2011; Roy 2010).

In parallel, then, it is now time to also ask solid critical questions about how researchers place the burden of change for gender equality and health on individual (and certain) men's shoulders. I have already argued in chapters 2 and 4 that neoliberalism, globalization, and other social and historical forces shape the available range of masculinities that men choose from, enact, wrestle with, contest, and reconfigure. This is critical to consider because current root causes for HIV clearly reside in very complex structural inequalities, and this is why, at the outset of this chapter, I have argued for the inclusion of structural-level interventions (Dworkin & Ehrhardt 2007; Blankenship, Bray, & Merson 2000; Blankenship et al. 2006; Gupta et al. 2008; Kerrigan et al. 2006; Parker, Easton, & Klein 2000; Sumartojo et al. 2000) that press beyond "gender norm change" so that there is structural backing for the maintenance of changed ideas about masculinities and gender equality.

At the same time, some scholars might balk at the suggestion that men should be offered structural solutions, agreeing that neoliberalism, unemployment, residential segregation, policing practices, and race relations have shaped gender relations but worrying that men will take the power derived in structural interventions and use it to widen the gaps in power between women and men. This fear might not be completely misguided, according to a few researchers who find that when men's wealth increases in some contexts, some men increase their expenditures on alcohol and additional sexual partners, increasing their own and their female partners' risks (Mishra et al. 2007). Such findings might fuel arguments that a gendered power gap is what negatively shaped women's and men's health to begin with and thus that improving men's structural situation may expand inequalities between women and men. Therefore, these considerations urge HIV-prevention scholars to consider the necessity of a new generation of structural interventions that are gender transformative and work explicitly on minimizing inequality between women and men. Such programs must also consider the complex intersections in these programmatic endeavors among structure, agency, and constraint—all of which are a merger of classic sociological, feminist, global and public health questions—the critical junctures at which this book rests.

It is also clear that social science insights about relational analyses of gender (Connell 1987; McKay 1997)—whereby the simultaneity of masculinities and femininities is taken into account—are critical for HIV- and violence-prevention studies in the domestic and global realm. Acting on such insights would mean including men in women's empowerment programs in order to democratize relationships between women and men and garner men's support for improvements in women's community, social, and household power. The success of a relational approach to HIV can be understood through the example of female-initiated methods of HIV/STI protection such as the female condom. My colleague Joanne Mantell and I (Mantell et al. 2006) argued that men should be integrated into the female-initiated-methods (female condoms and microbicides) trajectory—from a product's initial development to its reach in the marketplace—to maximize the use of these methods as prevention options. For example, we challenged notions that it is always necessary to encourage women's empowerment through "covert use" of female condoms, which are under the control of women. A relational approach to HIV prevention can be very important for building relationship equality, communication between partners, and relationship trust and satisfaction. Pool and colleagues in 2000 in their study of men's reactions to the use of female-initiated methods in Western Uganda share a quotation from a man in a focus group: "We would like our partners to use these products openly, not secretly, because we are struggling together to eliminate AIDS. If they use those products secretly it means that they think that men want to keep AIDS in existence. And secrecy can cause some misunderstandings between partners" (Pool et al. 2000, 204).

The above example and findings in chapter 3 and chapter 4 examined the limitations of solely viewing women or men as the target population for intervention, and underscored the potential instead of embracing the relational nature of gender. Relational analysis would entail engaging heterosexually active women and men simultaneously in the same program and wrestling with notions of equality and health alongside one another. This would mean sitting with and working through the tensions and contradictions that emerge when we think about gender as relational and that have long consumed feminist thinking (Will men "take over" if they are included? Will women's empowerment be "diluted"? Will women's causes lose important resources? Will the harms to men in the gender order be framed as "equal" to the harms to women instead of a nuanced understanding of differential harms being retained?) (Flood 2007, 2011). A relational approach to gender relations is increasingly being applied to One Man Can (personal conversation, Dean Peacock). A relational approach, when applied in gender-transformative programs, can dampen common misperceptions and can help to minimize commonly held beliefs that engaging men "takes away" resources or benefits from women because men can and do work towards the transformation of gender relations for the sake of social justice and health (Dworkin 2013; Peacock 2013).

A relational approach can underscore the importance of offering simultaneous attention to issues related to gendered power/women's empowerment and the costs of masculinity to men. Such an approach can also minimize or prevent backlash narratives and the actions that can subsequently follow from the ideologies that undergird backlash when men struggle with a feared loss of power that comes with the advances sought by women through women's rights frameworks or in women's empowerment programming. And HIV- and violence-prevention researchers and practitioners need to underscore that not just women but also men are situated within broader social and economic contexts (globalization, neoliberalism, poverty-reduction-strategy approaches that followed structural adjustment, unemployment) that have meant difficult changes not just for women but for both women and men. This kind of relational approach can help men to hear and embrace messages about the need for improved health for both women and men and diminish the sense that women's gains result in losses for men—an attitude that has been found in the literature on gender relations domestically and globally (Dworkin et al. 2012; Kimmel 1996, 2000). Still, however, it is important not to diminish the important point that I have previously underscored in chapter 3 and that researchers make when they underscore the "value of all-male and all-female initiatives" because they "fill a particular role in providing 'safe' spaces for men and women to express worries, share their personal stories, and seek advice" (Pulerwitz et al. 2010).

All of the above comments point to how interdisciplinary teams within the fields of HIV and violence prevention that focus on masculinities, intersectionalities, women's empowerment, gender relations, and health are urgently needed. Working across the disciplines of sociology, public health, global health, epidemiology, medicine, psychology, political economy, and anthropology can help to create new forms of critical thinking such as those employed in an emerging field mentioned in chapter 1 known as "critical global health" (Biehl & Petryna 2013), which the current book partly fits into. This kind of work, when carried out with global health and public health teams, can ensure that masculinities are not reduced to universal or decontextualized notions of masculinity and that intervention options are sifted through in a multilevel and interdisciplinary manner. With or without these assurances, another question remains: what are gender-transformative interventions really transforming?

"Being a Better Man": Masculinity and Structural Change in Gender-Transformative Health Programming

Recall from chapter 1 that while there are limitations to focusing on "gender roles" and "gender norms" in the HIV epidemic, recognition of gender roles and norms among men in the HIV epidemic advanced the field by recognizing the dynamic nature of social interactions and the concept that gender is "done" (West & Zimmerman 1987; West & Fenstermaker 1995) and can be "undone." As I mentioned in chapters 1–4, if in HIV prevention the route to reducing HIV risk is to insist that gender norms should just be "done differently," then this can lead to a lack of recognition of the structural/institutional and historically patterned nature of gender relations, which are also inflected by race, class, and sexuality relations. Also recall that the men referred to in chapter 4 saw the benefits of reconfiguring masculine practice and saw themselves as active agents in the gender order. Unfortunately, as I have reiterated throughout this book, very little HIV-related work is gender transformative in the United States, and even fewer studies are structurally informed (for one exception, see Raj et al. 2013).

In earlier parts of the book and in this chapter, I have argued that the analytical move to a focus on gender-norm transformation within the field of HIV prevention often uncritically pins together the parts of the sex-gender-sexuality triad. The assumptions that undergird a sex-gender-sexuality triad in HIV prevention largely emphasize that people who were born male will socially enact *one* gender role (that of hegemonic masculinity, even though the men who are targeted in HIV prevention are largely subordinated by race and class status)—and gender was often uncritically pinned to an assumed heterosexuality (even though there can be disjunctures between sexual acts and identities for heterosexually identified men). In South Africa in particular, part of the assumption of 100% heterosexuality in the science base is certainly due to homophobia and the fact that same-sex sexuality was criminalized during apartheid (Gevisser & Cameron 1995; Hoad 2005; Hoad, Martin, & Reid 2005). After the official end of apartheid, despite the fact that South Africa was the first country in the world to include gays and lesbians in its constitution as having rights that are deserving of the protection and support afforded full citizens (Munro 2012; Swarr 2012), there are enormous challenges to fully recognizing gays, lesbians, bisexuals, and transgendered populations—and homophobia has played a large role in preventing marginalized sexualities from becoming more visible and in preventing a full-scale response to marginalized sexualities in the HIV epidemic (Reddy, Sandfort, & Rispel 2010).

In fact, assumptions that the epidemic is largely "heterosexual" in South Africa—and that there is a "heterosexual epidemic" in the United States—further mask the fact that many men might identify as heterosexual but have sex with men or both women and men (Dodge et al. 2012; Epprecht 2008, 2013; Reddy, Sandfort, & Rispel 2011). Looking at South Africa in particular, the history and contemporary state of male-male and GLBT sexualities in South Africa have been excavated in detail by anthropologists, historians, women's studies scholars, public- and global-health scholars, and within numerous other disciplines (Donham 1998; Epprecht 2008, 2013; Gevisser & Cameron 1995; Moodie, Ndatse, & Sibuyi 1998; Niehaus 2009; Reddy, Sandfort, & Rispel 2010; Swarr 2012). Thus, it is clear that all gender-transformative programming can do a more thorough job of asking meticulous questions about whether a man's sexual partners are male, female, or transgender. Doing so will cause public health workers to think more carefully about the ways in which "gender transformation" may need modification to impact HIV risks with various partners. In addition, there is much room for future prevention work to introduce the benefits of queer theory from sociology and other disciplines (Halberstam 2005; Namaste 1994; Somervillle 2000; Turner 2000; Valocchi 2007; Warner 1993) to further challenge the all-too-common connections made between elements of the sex-gender-sexuality triad in HIV prevention both domestically and globally. This is a ripe area for future research. There is also an opportunity for future work to apply the insights derived from masculinities-based work to the study of reducing HIV risk among men who have sex with men.

I have pointed to the possibility that gender-transformative work can have the inadvertent consequence of calling upon men to change their ideals of masculinity that are being indirectly (or, some might argue, directly) blamed for inequality and health problems. Indeed, there are broader interdisciplinary critiques of gender-transformative work that are possible and are worth considering. For example, postcolonial and/or globalization scholars might argue that the call for men to shift masculinities on their own absolves the state and transnational relations from improving the structural conditions of its own citizens in ways that can positively shape health (Castle 2001; Hunter 2005). That is, to ask Black men in South Africa to change when masculinities have been shaped under the heinous conditions of an apartheid and colonial history and now a postcolonial and neoliberal state erases the fact that these very circumstances helped to structure the range of masculinities that men choose from and are constrained into. From this perspective, when global health scholars deploy methods of individual and community norm change in gender-transformative programs, they may be bolstering a neoliberal view of society. Such a view shifts responsibility for one's health onto citizens without adequately responding to racism, classism, and an oppressive gender order in ways that help citizens to make health and equality more possible to achieve (Hunter 2005; Lupton 1995). Along these lines, men's narratives of "being a new man" might say less about becoming gender equitable and more about becoming a certain kind of "healthy" citizen: redemptive, changed, self-regulating.

Of interest, there are also a variety of religious scholars in South Africa and elsewhere in sub-Saharan Africa who focus on "redemptive masculinities" (Chitando & Chirongoma 2012) wherein creative evangelism is used to "produce a social space where dominant masculinities are disrupted and contradicted and where alternatives can be articulated that lead, potentially, to social transformation" (van Klinken 2013b, 287). It is critical to point out that the idea systems that undergird redemptive-masculinities (to reduce HIV and violence) and gender-transformative work are somewhat similar. Scholars in the area of redemptive masculinities agree with gender-transformative researchers that masculinities are constructed, that race and class relations shape the historical specificity of masculinities, and that it is possible to positively engage men in combating HIV and violence (Chitando & Chirongoma 2012; Isike & Okeke-Uzodike 2008; van Klinken 2013a, 2013b). Both redemptive and gender-transformative approaches are critical of overdetermined notions of powerless women and powerful men and recognize the plurality of masculinities. Both approaches recognize the historical influence of colonialism, poverty, and race relations in shaping social constructions of masculinities, and accordingly, the historical specificity of and contextual influences on masculinity are at the forefront of ideas about how to intervene. In both approaches, men are engaged in re-envisioning masculinities so that these are not harmful to health and in reconfiguring the norms and practices that lead to new health practices. In both approaches, men who are "gender-friendly" are encouraged to be role models to other men, showing them how to make positive changes in health practices. And, lastly, shared parenting and shared gendered divisions of household labor are viewed in both types of programs as ways to increase equality between men and women.

Two main differences separate some of the religious writings on redemptive masculinity and gender-transformative work. First, several of the religious writings argued that precolonial men were more egalitarian in gender relations, that men have been warped by colonial notions of inferiority and superiority, and that if men recognized this, then they would understand that male dominance is not natural but constructed and can be changed. In addition, such writings emphasize how African notions of collectivism are at odds with neoliberal conceptions of individualism, and if African men returned to their "African roots," then they would engage notions of sharing and caring more. While many of the religious writings show sophistication in their coverage of masculinities and are potentially helpful in shifting notions of masculinity, some of these ideas seem to uncritically assume that there is an essen-

tial African man who should return to his "true" "roots" and personhood, an idea that has been challenged by postcolonial thinkers and
social scientists alike. Second, despite the call for men to share child
care and household labor in the redemptive masculinities literature,
there is less of an emphasis on seeking equitable relationships between
men and women overall and more of an emphasis on maintaining men
as heads of households. These differences in thinking are due to the
fact that redemptive masculinities scholars retain a belief in male and
female differences that are viewed as God-given or biologically created
(van Klinken 2011, 2013a, 2013b).

What is unclear in the redemptive-masculinity stance is how such
an approach would impact HIV risks. How might this programming
reinforce notions of male dominance in some arenas while undermining
it in other realms? Because this approach states that it recognizes that
gender inequality and the costs of masculinity negatively impact health
but simultaneously reinforces male-dominated decision making in certain realms, it is not clear what the impacts of this particular approach
would be on gender equality or health outcomes. Such approaches need
testing in the science base and could prove to be interesting projects,
just as gender-sensitive approaches in the United States that recognize
gendered power have been modified to intervene on HIV risks in the
lives of African American women who have very strong faith-related
beliefs and attend Black mega-churches (Wingood et al. 2013; Wingood,
Simpson-Robinson, et al. 2013).

Also consider that despite the social-justice emphasis in gender-
transformative programs, these programs ask some men to change their
manhood while White middle-class and more privileged heterosexually
active men are not under the public/global health gaze and are therefore
not asked to change their notions of masculinities in order to be "better
men." As has been argued by Moffett (2008) when she refers to South
African society as "battling to shake off the legacy of institutionalized
racism" and underscores that

> it still seems a bridge too far to acknowledge that gender is at the heart
> of this acute social problem [violence]. Instead one hears repeatedly that
> apartheid and its ills (such as the migrant labor system) "emasculated"
> black men, left them "impotent" and experiencing a "crisis of masculin-

ity." Though these remarks are troublingly embedded in unquestioned patriarchal discourses . . . these explanations explicitly exclude White men thus implying—however unwittingly—that they do not rape [or transmit HIV]. (111)

In short, while it is clearly not an overt goal in either gender-transformative or redemptive-masculinities approaches to do so, perhaps both approaches might inadvertently and indirectly bolster notions of violent and sexually "excessive" race- and class-marginalized men (who are being told they need to change), unknowingly reinforcing inequalities among men (Dworkin & Messner 1999) within nations and between men from different nations.

What is so critical to keep in mind about the One Man Can Program and the kind of citizenship that it engenders is this: it does put forward a partly individualizing public health message that places changing masculinities and engaging new health behaviors on men's shoulders, but it also includes a sense of *individual and social/collective responsibility* for changing gender inequality and reshaping violence and HIV risks. Embedded within an NGO, this program is certainly influenced by public health and the state, as President Mbeki has reportedly "made it clear" that "when it came to AIDS, the stakes were far higher than simply the issue of the nation's physical health; its ethical well-being, and the integrity of its social and political body, were similarly at risk" (Posel 2008, 22). However, the program I examined was not firmly located within the government nor the public health enterprise but rather is offered by a nongovernmental organization that is committed to radically transforming society through social activism and advocacy of human rights in the area of gender and sexuality relations. It would therefore be impossible to fully understand the content of One Man Can or its strategies or impacts—or the men's narratives covered in chapter 4—without offering brief coverage of the role of nongovernmental organizations in shaping local social movements and health programs in postapartheid South Africa.

Robins has examined social movements, NGOs, rights, and political action during and after apartheid in South Africa and is particularly skilled in this regard (2008a, 2008b). He argues that in fact NGOs engage in and constitute complex social processes that are important to unpack in attempts to understand their missions, practices, and impacts. He argues that many NGOs in South Africa should not simply be viewed as handmaidens to the state that reinforce docile citizen subjects but rather should be understood to operate as NGO–social movement partnerships that "have contributed towards expanding conventional conceptions of civil society, rights, and citizenship" (Robins 2008a, 21). He argues that in a society where large numbers of people are living on the margins and are disenfranchised, it is very difficult for the state to garner loyalty from its citizens. This is the case even though South Africa cannot be viewed as a neoliberal economy only, because it also has large social grant programs that reach over twelve million people in a population of fifty million and does emphasize communitarian principles in several of its policies (Colvin, Robins, & Leavens 2010). However, as I mentioned in chapter 4, despite its progressive constitution and its attempts to help the vast masses of poor people who are disproportionately Black, the Black unemployment rates remain abominably high, rates of poverty are extremely high, and the nation ranks number one in unequal distribution of income. Thus, "because of these limitations of the post-apartheid liberal democratic state," it is NGOs, new social movements, and other thriving and dynamic civil society responses that have stepped in to respond to failures in the areas of housing, jobs, land, poverty, and, as we have seen, violence and HIV/AIDS program (Colvin, Robins, & Leavens 2010).

Thus, while in a variety of literatures, including the development and feminist literatures, NGOs have been criticized as being too close to the state or as weakening feminist issues through professional accountability practices that are found within state institutions, it is critical to keep in mind that these types of analyses lose sight of the subjectivities, agency, collective action, and positive consequences that can arise from NGO programs. Indeed, Robins argues that NGOs, in conjunction with social movements (such as feminist social movements in the case of Sonke), help to intervene not only in health-related issues but also in issues of anomie, social isolation, and feelings of uselessness that have emerged in the broader context of intensive poverty, neoliberalism, and structural instabilities.

Recall that the men in the first sample described in chapter 4 frequently mentioned that they felt useless, disconnected, disrespected, and unproductive, particularly when unemployed. Thus, while rampant globalization and consumerism, neoliberalism, and poverty can appear to many to "be the only games in town" in South Africa, NGOs have increasingly "played a critical role at the juncture of rights, solidarity, sociality, and social transformation" (Robins 2008a, 21) that cannot be so easily discounted. Additionally, scholars have argued extensively about the ways in which the transition to democracy in South Africa involved the nation becoming a specifically gendered state in many new ways (that were described in chapter 4) due to the work of numerous feminist groups, lobbyists, and activists (Kemp et al. 1995; Seidman 1999). These groups, with much influence from Black South African women, demanded that a "nonracial, democratic, non-sexist" state emerge through gendered representation, policies, and the formation of numerous organizations that were funded with international donor money to advance women's rights (Seidman 1999).

To be clear, then, Sonke Gender Justice emerged in this context of neoliberal imperatives, a populace increasingly frustrated with the state, and increasing donor funds used to form NGO organizations that assist with the development of a burgeoning democracy that presses for government accountability. Pressing for government accountability is central to the work that Sonke does. Thus, it should be no surprise that the One Man Can program was launched on International Day to End Violence in 2006 in South Africa and then in Geneva on December 6, 2006. It was launched as a formal partnership with a wide variety of South African, women's rights, and international organizations that seek not just to support the rights of marginalized populations but to achieve governmental change.

The number of NGOs in South Africa most certainly did exponentially increase in a context of globalization and neoliberalism that led to a retracted state. As a result, it is certainly possible to interpret gender-transformative programming, in the words of Hardt and Negri (2000), as a "moral intervention" being offered by NGOs who (these authors think) are all in service of global capitalism and are being used to bolster the political order associated with globalization. However, rather than being in service to global capitalism, it is clear that Sonke Gender Justice spends much of its time challenging state policies. Sonke labors to hold government accountable to its promises to work to end gendered and sexual violence, as well as rape and torture in prisons, to improve national HIV policies, and to promote the engagement of men in policy efforts to end violence against women and reduce the spread of HIV. Thus, I prefer to understand NGOs such as the one I've studied and its strategy of gender-transformative work as being in partnership with social movements that "secure access to state resources by deploying both local rights-based strategies and globally connected modes of collective mobilization in marginalized communities" (Robins 2008a, 5). Thus, I see the One Man Can program as Appadurai (2001) would when he refers to a trend towards globalization that is grassroots, or from below. One Man Can reveals the dynamics of globalization from below, which emphasizes feminist-inspired "new forms of community participation and citizenship" (Robins 2008a, 142) and "new masculinities and identities" that are "very much in the making" (Robins 2008a, 161).

Some readers will see the results in this book as evidence of feminist victories, and some will remain unconvinced. Some might argue that gender-transformative interventions may be rife with talk of individual responsibility for becoming more egalitarian and healthy that is infused with "a hierarchy of action, in which self-care and responsibility for one's health are at the top" (Lupton 1995, 53) (as is often the case in public health programming). This can certainly serve to marginalize or stigmatize marginalized groups who are considered to be unhealthy or "risky" (Lupton 1995). Simultaneously, however, we can see from the men's narratives presented in chapter 4 that they did not express a sense of moralized oppression or an overwhelming sense that rights were an intrusion into their lives and homes that was being imposed from the West in an unwelcome manner. Rather, they were aware of their chronic poverty, had strong recognition of the ways they were experiencing structural unemployment, and bemoaned their inability to secure a wife or pay *lobola* (monetary exchange a man makes to the bride's family). Men were acutely aware of government calls for "50–50" and described new configurations of gendered power and practice— and they wrestled with how to apply these in their sexual relationships, homes, and communities.

Thus men described old and new engagement with ideas about gendered power and the ways to apply rights-based discourses to their lives. They tried on new notions of masculinities and identities and enacted new modes of caring for themselves and others. They described new modes of mobilization where they actively and agentically fought for gendered social change as defined by a combination of local needs, a thriving civil society and human rights culture, and a need for social solidarity that was coupled with a desire to press beyond feeling "useless." Men talked about "sharing important things" with their partners about sexuality, decision making, household labor, safe sex, and HIV and AIDS. Men talked about how they had conversations with other men on the topics of violence, HIV prevention, HIV treatment, and sharing household labor and power.

In this way, men in our study articulated what Colvin, Robins, and Leavens (2010) might call new forms of "responsibilized citizenship" that are not only individual but immanently *social* and are coupled with what Nguyen (2005) might call new modes of caring about oneself, one's sexual partners, and one's family and community. And while some may be unsure whether NGOs in South Africa or the content in gender-transformative HIV programming more broadly reinforces "docile and disciplined subjects" or produces a new form of "responsible, empowered, and knowledgeable citizens" (Robins 2008a, 164), one thing is certain: gender-transformative work has shifted the field of HIV and violence prevention and is one small step closer to intersectional HIV/AIDS- and violence-prevention programming that will be designed in the future. One day, science-based content and NGO work in these substantive areas will conceive of these two synergistic and profoundly important epidemics (violence and HIV/AIDS) as defined by intersectional structural inequalities—and intersectional identities—and the prevention solutions will be conceived of accordingly. That next generation of work may very well make a more lasting imprint on reducing violence and HIV risks both domestically and globally. The health of men and women depends on it.

REFERENCES

Action Aids International (2006). The impact of girls' education on HIV and sexual behavior: Girl power. Education and HIV Series 101. Accessed on February 8, 2012, at http://www.ungei.org/resources/files/girl_power_2006.pdf

Adimora, A. A., Schoenbach, V. J., & Floris-Moore, M. A. (2009). Ending the epidemic of heterosexual HIV transmission among African Americans. *American Journal of Preventive Medicine, 37*, 468–71.

Adimora A. A., Schoenbach, V. J., Martinson, F., Donaldson, K. H., Stancil, T. R., & Fullilove, R. E. (2004). Concurrent sexual partnerships among African Americans in the rural south. *Annals of Epidemiology, 14*, 155–60.

Adimora, A. A., et al. (2003). Concurrent partnerships among rural African Americans with recently reported heterosexual infection. *Journal of Acquired Immune Deficiency Syndromes, 34*, 423–29.

Aidala, A., et al. (2005). Housing status and HIV risk behaviors: Implications for prevention and policy. *AIDS & Behavior, 9*, 251–65.

Al-Amin, M., & Chowdhury, T. (2008). Women, poverty, and empowerment: An investigation into the dark side of microfinance. *Asian Affairs, 30*, 6–29.

Albert, S. (2001). Many lesbian and bisexual women unaware of risks. *Gay Health.* Available at http://www.gayhealth.com/iowa-robot/sex/?record=407

Alcamo, I. E. (2002). *AIDS in the Modern World.* Malden, MA: Blackwell Science.

Almaguer, T. (1990). Chicano men: A cartography of homosexual identity and behavior. Pp. 255–74 in H. Abelove (ed.), *The Lesbian and Gay Studies Reader.* New York: Routledge.

Altbeker, A. (2007). *A Country at War with Itself: South Africa's Crisis of Crime.* Johannesburg: Jonathan Bell Publishers.

Altman, D. (2000). Sex and Political Economy. Paper presented at the Ford Foundation Workshop on Sexuality and Social Change: An Agenda for Research and Action in the 21st Century, Rio de Janeiro.

Amaro, H. (1995). Love, sex, and power: Considering women's realities in HIV prevention. *American Psychologist, 50*, 437–47.

Amaro, H., Blake, S., Schwartz, P. M., and Flinchbaugh, L. J. (2001). Developing theory-based substance-abuse prevention programs for young adolescent girls. *Journal of Early Adolescence, 21*, 256–93.

Amaro, H., Raj, A., & Reed, E. (2001). Women's sexual health: The need for feminist analyses in public health in the decade of behavior. *Psychology of Women Quarterly, 25*, 324–34.

Anderson, R. M., May, R. M., Boily, M. C., Garnett, G. P., & Rowley, J. T. (1991). The spread of HIV-1 in Africa: Sexual contact patterns and the predicted demographic impact of AIDS. *Nature, 352,* 581–90.

Anema, A., Vogenthaler, N., Frongillo, E. A., Kadiyala, S., & Weiser, S. D. (2009). Food insecurity and HIV/AIDS: Current knowledge, gaps, and research priorities. *Current HIV/AIDS Reports, 6,* 224–31.

Anzaldua, G., Cantu, L., & Hertado, A. (2012). *Borderlands/La Frontera: The New Mestiza* (4th ed). San Francisco: Aunt Lute Books.

Appadurai, A. (2001). *Globalization.* Durham, NC: Duke University Press.

Auerbach, J., & Adimora, A. (2010). Structural interventions for HIV prevention in the United States. *Journal of Acquired Immune Deficiency Syndromes, 55,* S132–35.

Baca-Zinn, M., & Thornton-Dill, B. (1993). Difference and domination. Pp. 3–12 in M. Baca Zinn & B. Thornton-Dill (eds.), *Women of Color in U.S. Society.* Philadelphia: Temple University Press.

Baker, S. A., Beadnell, B., Stoner, S., et al. (2004). Skills training versus health education to prevent STDs/HIV in heterosexual women: A randomized controlled trial utilizing biological outcomes. *AIDS Education & Prevention, 15,* 1–14.

Barker G. (2000). Department of Child and Adolescent Health, World Health Organization. *What about Boys? A Literature Review on the Health and Development of Adolescent Boys.* Geneva, Switzerland: World Health Organization.

Barker, G. (2005). *Dying to Be Men: Youth, Masculinity, and Social Exclusion.* New York: Routledge.

Barker, G. (2008). Promoting gender equity as a strategy to reduce HIV risk and gender-based violence among young men in India. Washington, DC: Population Council. Available at http://www.popcouncil.org/pdfs/horizons/India_Gender-Norms.pdf

Barker, G., Ricardo, C., & Nascimento, M. (2007). *Engaging Men and Boys in Changing Gender-Based Inequity in Health: Evidence from Programme Interventions.* Geneva, Switzerland: World Health Organization. Available at http://www.who.int/gender/documents/Engaging_men_boys.pdf

Barker, G., Ricardo, C., Nascimento, M., Olukoya, A., & Santos C. (2010). Questioning gender norms with men to improve health outcomes: Evidence of impact. *Global Public Health, 5,* 539–53.

Barker, G., & Schulte, J. (2010). Engaging men as allies in women's economic empowerment: Strategies and recommendations for CARE country offices. Available online.

Barry, A., Osborne, T., & Rose, N. (eds.) (1996). *Foucault and Practical Reason: Liberalism, Neoliberalism, and Rationalities of Government.* London: University College London.

Beadnell, B., Baker, S., Morrison, D. M., & Knox, K. (2000). HIV/STD risk factors for women with violent male partners. *Sex Roles, 42,* 661–89.

Bentley, K. (2004). Women's rights and the feminization of poverty in South Africa. *Review of African Political Economy, 100,* 247–61.

Berer, M. (1993). *Women and AIDS: An International Resource Book.* London: HarperCollins.

Berger, M. (2005). *Workable Sisterhood: The Political Journey of Stigmatized Women with HIV/AIDS*. Princeton, NJ: Princeton University Press.

Bernstein, E. (2010). Militarized humanitarianism meets carceral feminism: The politics of sex, rights, and freedom in contemporary anti-trafficking campaigns. *SIGNS: Journal of Women in Culture and Society, 36*, 46–71.

Bevier, P. J., Chiasson, M. A., Heffernan, R. T., & Castro, K. G. (1995). Women at a sexually transmitted disease clinic: Their HIV seroprevalence and risk behaviors. *American Journal of Public Health, 85*, 1366–76.

Biehl, J., & Petryna, A. (eds.) (2013). *When People Come First: Critical Studies in Global Health*. Princeton, NJ: Princeton University Press.

Bingham, T. A., Harawa, N. T., Johnson, D. F., Secura, G. M., Mackellar, D. A., & Valleroy, L. A. (2003). The effect of partner characteristics on HIV infection among African-American men who have sex with men in the Young Men's Survey, Los Angeles, 1999–2000. *AIDS Education & Prevention, 15*, 39–52.

Blankenship K., Bray, S. J., & Merson, M. H. (2000). Structural interventions in public health. *AIDS, 14* (Supplement 1), S11–S21.

Blankenship, K. M., Friedman, S. R., Dworkin, S., & Mantell, J. E. (2006). Structural interventions: Concepts, challenges, and opportunities for research. *Journal of Urban Health, 83*, 59–72.

Blumstein, P., & Schwartz, P. (1983). *American Couples: Money, Work, Sex*. New York: Morrow.

Bond, P. (2000). *Elite Transition: From Apartheid to Neoliberalism in South Africa*. London: Pluto.

Boonzaier, E., & Spiegel, A. D. (2008). Tradition. Pp. 195–208 in N. Shepherd & S. Robins (eds.), *New South African Keywords*. Athens: Ohio University Press.

Bornstein, D. (2013). Beyond Profit: A Talk with Muhammad Yunus. *New York Times*, April 17, 2013. Available at http://opinionator.blogs.nytimes.com/2013/04/17/beyond-profit-a-talk-with-muhammad-yunus/?ref=microfinance&_r=0

Bowleg, L. (2004). Love, sex, and masculinity in sociocultural context. *Men and Masculinities, 7*, 166–86.

Bowleg, L. (2012). The problem with the phrase women and minorities: Intersectionality—an important theoretical framework for public health. *American Journal of Public Health, 102*, 1267–73.

Bowleg, L., & Raj, A. (2012). Shared communities, structural contexts, and HIV risk: Prioritizing the HIV risk and prevention needs of Black heterosexual men. *American Journal of Public Health, 102*, S173–77.

Bowleg, L., et al. (2011). What does it take to be a man: What is a real man; Ideologies of masculinity and HIV risk among black heterosexual men. *Culture, Health, & Sexuality, 13*, 545–59.

Brett, J. A. (2006). We sacrifice and we eat less: The structural complexities of microfinance participation. *Human Organization, 65*, 8–19.

Brod, H. (1988). Pornography and the alienation of male sexuality. *Social Theory and Practice, 14*, 265–84.

Brod, H. (1995). Pornography and the alienation of male sexuality. Pp. 393–404 in Michael Kimmel & Michael A. Messner (eds.), *Men's Lives*. Boston: Allyn & Bacon

Butler, J. (1993). *Bodies That Matter: On the Discursive Limits of Sex*. New York: Taylor & Francis.

Byers, E. S. (1996). How well does the traditional sexual script explain sexual coercion? Review of a program of research. Pp. 7–26 in E. Sandra Byers & Lucia O'Sullivan (eds.), *Sexual Coercion in Dating Relationships*. New York: Haworth Press.

Camlin, C., Kwena, Z., & Dworkin, S. L. (2013). *Jaboya* vs. *Jakambi*: Status, negotiation, and HIV risks among female migrants in the "sex for fish" trade in Nyanza Province, Kenya. *AIDS Education & Prevention, 25*, 216–31.

Campbell, C. (1995). Male gender roles and sexuality: Implications for women's AIDS risk and prevention. *Social Science and Medicine, 41*, 97–210.

Campbell, C. (1999). *Women, Families, and the HIV Epidemic: A Sociological Perspective on the Epidemic in America*. New York: Cambridge University Press.

Campos, P., Saguy, A., Ernsberger, P., Oliver, E., & Gaesser, G. (2006). The epidemiology of overweight and obesity: Public health crisis or moral panic? *International Journal of Epidemiology, 35*, 55–60.

Canetto, S. S. (1995). Men who survive a suicidal act. Pp. 292–304 in D. Sabo & D. F. Gordon (eds.), *Men's Health and Illness: Gender, Power, and the Body*. New York: Sage.

Carael, M. (1995). Sexual behaviour. Pp. 75–123 in J. Cleland & B. Ferry (eds.), *Sexual Behavior and AIDS in the Developing World: Findings from a Multisite Study*. London: Taylor and Francis.

Carey, M. P., Carey, K. B., Maisto, S. A., et al. (2004). Reducing HIV risk behavior among adults receiving outpatient psychiatric treatment: Results from a randomized controlled trial. *Journal of Consulting and Clinical Psychology, 72*, 252–68.

Carrillo, H. (2002). *The Night Is Young: Sexuality in Mexico in the Time of AIDS*. Chicago: University of Chicago Press.

Castle, G. (2001). *Postcolonial Discourses: An Anthology*. Oxford: Blackwell.

Cawthorne, A. (2010). Poverty is driving an HIV epidemic: CDC study shows that combating HIV means combating poverty. Available at www.americanprogress.org/issues/poverty/news/2010/07/21/8101/poverty-is-driving-an-hiv-epidemic

Centers for Disease Control and Prevention (CDC) (1992). 1993 revised classification system for HIV infection and expanded surveillance case definition for AIDS among adolescents and adults. *Morbidity Mortality Weekly Report, 41*, 17.

Centers for Disease Control and Prevention (CDC) (1995). Update: AIDS among women in the United States, 1994. *Morbidity Mortality Weekly Report, 44*, 81–84.

Centers for Disease Control and Prevention (CDC) (2000). HIV/AIDS and U.S. women who have sex with women (WSW). Available at http://www.cdc.gov/hiv/pubs/facts/wsw.html

Centers for Disease Control and Prevention (CDC) (2002a). AIDS cases in adolescents and adults by age—United States, 1994–2000. *HIV/AIDS Surveillance Supplemental Report, 9* (1).

Centers for Disease Control and Prevention (CDC) (2002b). Cases of HIV infection and AIDS in the United States, 2002. Available at http://stacks.cdc.gov/view/cdc/5677/Share.

Centers for Disease Control and Prevention (CDC) (2011). Mortality slide series. Available at http://www.cdc.gov/hiv/library/slideSets/index.html

Centers for Disease Control and Prevention (CDC) (2012). Estimated HIV incidence among adults and adolescents in the United States, 2007–2010. *HIV Surveillance Supplemental Report, 17* (4).

Centers for Disease Control and Prevention (CDC) (2013a). HIV Surveillance: Epidemiology of HIV infection. Available at http://www.cdc.gov/hiv/pdf/g-l/cdc-hiv-genepislideseries-2013.pdf

Centers for Disease Control and Prevention (CDC) (2013b). Epidemiology of HIV infection through 201. Available at http://www.cdc.gov/hiv/library/slideSets/index.html

Centers for Disease Control and Prevention (CDC) (2013c). HIV/AIDS surveillance by race/ethnicity. Available at http://www.cdc.gov/hiv/pdf/HIV_2013_RaceEthnicitySlides_508.pdf

Centers for Disease Control and Prevention (CDC) (2013d). Mortality slide series. Available at http://www.cdc.gov/hiv/library/slideSets/index.html

Centers for Disease Control and Prevention (CDC) (2013e). HIV Surveillance in Women. Available at http://www.cdc.gov/hiv/pdf/q-z/cdc-hiv-surveillance-in-women-2013.pdf

Centers for Disease Control and Prevention (CDC) (2013f). Condom distribution as a structural intervention. Available at http://www.cdc.gov/hiv/prevention/programs/condoms/index.html

Centers for Disease Control and Prevention (CDC) (2014). HIV among African Americans. Available at http://www.cdc.gov/hiv/pdf/HIV-AA-english-508.pdf

Cheemeh, P. E., Montoya, I. D., Essien, E. J., & Ogungbade, G. O. (2006). HIV/AIDS in the Middle East: A guide to a proactive response. *Journal of the Royal Society for the Promotion of Health, 126,* 165–71.

Chitando, E., & Chirongoma, S. (eds.) (2012). *Redemptive Masculinities: Men, HIV, and Religion.* Geneva, Switzerland: WCC Publications. Available online.

Chodorow, N. (1978). *The Reproduction of Mothering: Psychoanalysis and the Sociology of Gender.* Berkeley: University of California Press.

Choi, K. H., & Coates, T. J. (1994). Prevention of HIV infection. *AIDS, 8,* 1371–89.

Choi, K. H., Rickman, R., & Catania, J. A. (1994). What heterosexual adults believe about condoms. *New England Journal of Medicine, 331,* 406–7.

Cock, J. (2005). Engendering gay and lesbian rights: The equality clause in the South African Constitution. Pp. 188–89 in N. Hoad, K. Martin, & G. Reid (eds.), *Sex and Politics in South Africa.* Cape Town: Double Storey Books.

Cohan, N., & Atwood, J. D. (1994). Women and AIDS: The social construction of gender and diseases. *Family Systems Medicine, 12,* 5–20.

Cole, E. R. (2009). Intersectionality and research in psychology. *American Psychologist, 64*, 170–180. Available at http://sitemaker.umich.edu/cole.qsort/files/cole_intersectionality_in_psych.pdf

Colvin, C. (2011). Executive summary report on the impact of Sonke Gender Justice's One Man Can Campaign in Limpopo, Eastern Cape, and Kwa-Zulu Natal, South Africa. Available at www.genderjustice.org.za.

Colvin, C., Robins, S., & Leavens, J. (2010). Grounding "responsibilization" talk: Masculinities, citizenship, and HIV in Cape Town, South Africa. *Journal of Development Studies, 46*, 1179–95.

Conley, T. D., & Collins, B. E. (2005). Differences between condom users and condom nonusers in their multidimensional condom attitudes. *Journal of Applied Social Psychology, 35*, 603–20.

Connell, R. W. (1987). *Gender & Power: Society, the Person, and Sexual Politics.* Palo Alto, CA: Stanford University Press.

Connell, R. W. (1995a). *Masculinities.* Berkeley: University of California Press.

Connell, R. W. (1995b). Masculinity, violence, and war. In Michael S. Kimmel & Michael A. Messner (eds.), *Men's Lives.* Boston: Allyn & Bacon.

Connell, R. W., & Dowsett, G. (1999). The unclean motion of the generative parts: Frameworks in Western thought on sexuality. Pp. 449–72 in R. Parker & P. Aggleton (eds.), *Culture, Society, and Sexuality: A Reader.* Philadelphia: Taylor & Francis.

Connell, R. W., & Messerschmidt, J. W. (2005). Hegemonic masculinity. *Gender & Society, 19*, 829–59.

Cooky, C., & Dworkin, S. L. (2013). Policing the boundaries of sex: A critical examination of gender verification and the Caster Semenya controversy. *Journal of Sex Research, 50*, 103–11.

Courtenay, W. H. (2000a). Behavioral factors associated with disease, injury, and death among men: Evidence and implications for prevention. *Journal of Men's Studies, 9*, 81–129.

Courtenay, W. H. (2000b). Constructions of masculinity and their influence on men's well-being: A theory of gender and health. *Social Science & Medicine, 50*, 1385–1401.

Courtenay, W. H. (2000c). Engendering health: A social constructionist examination of men's health beliefs and behaviors. *Psychology of Men and Masculinity, 1*, 4–15.

Crawford, J., Kippax, S., & Waldby, C. (1994).Women's sex talk and men's sex talk: Different worlds. *Feminism & Psychology, 4*, 571–87.

Crawford, R. (1980). Healthism and the medicalization of everyday life. *International Journal of Health Services, 7*, 663–80.

Crenshaw, K. W. (1991). Mapping the margins: Intersectionality, identity politics, and violence against women of color. *Stanford Law Review, 43*, 1241–99.

Crosby, R., Holtgrave, D. R., Stall, R., Peterson, J. L., & Shouse, L. (2007). Differences in HIV risk behaviors among black and white men who have sex with men. *Sexually Transmitted Disease, 34*, 744–48.

Crosset, T. (2000). Athletic affiliation and violence against women: Towards a structural prevention project. Pp. 147–61 in J. McKay, D. F. Sabo, & M. A. Messner (eds.), *Masculinities, Gender Relations, and Sport*. Thousand Oaks, CA: Sage.

Crosset, T. W., Benedict, J. R., McDonald, M. (1995). Male student-athletes reported for sexual assaults: A survey of campus police departments and judicial affairs offices. *Journal of Sport and Social Issues, 19*, 126–40.

Curry, T. (1991). Fraternal bonding in the locker room: Pro-feminist analysis of talk about competition and women. *Sociology of Sport Journal, 9*, 119–35.

Darling, C. A., Davidson, J. K. Sr., & Conway-Welch, C. (1990). Female ejaculation, perceived origins, the Grafenberg spot/area, and sexual responsiveness. *Archives of Sexual Behavior, 19*, 29–47.

David, D. S., & Brannon, R. (1976). *The Forty-Nine Percent Majority: The Male Sex Role*. Boston: Addison Wesley.

DeLamater, J., & Hyde, J. (2007). *Understanding Human Sexuality*. New York: McGraw-Hill.

Delius, P., & Glaser, C. (2002). Sexual socialization in South Africa: A historical perspective. *African Studies, 61*, 27–54.

Denning, P., & DiNenno, E. (2010). Communities in crisis: Is there a generalized epidemic in impoverished urban areas of the United States? Available at http://origin. glb.cdc.gov/hiv/risk/other/poverty.html

Department of Health, South Africa (2012). Available at http://www.doh.gov.za.

de Walque, D. (2006). Discordant couples: HIV infection among couples in Burkina Faso, Cameroon, Ghana, Kenya, and Tanzania. Policy Research Working Paper: The World Bank. Report no. WPS3956. Available online.

Diaz, R. M. (1998). *Latino Gay Men and HIV: Culture, Sexuality, and Risk Behavior*. New York Routledge.

DiClemente, R., Wingood, G. M., Harrington, K. F., et al. (2004). Efficacy of an HIV prevention intervention for African American adolescent girls. *JAMA, 292*, 171–79.

Dodge, B., Jeffries, W. L., & Sandfort, T. G. M. (2008). Beyond the down low: Sexual risk, protection, and disclosure among at-risk Black men who have sex with men and women (MSMW). *Archives of Sexual Behavior, 37*, 683–96.

Dodge, B., Reece, M., & Gebhard, P. H. (2008). Kinsey & beyond: Past, present, & future considerations for research on male bisexuality. *Journal of Bisexuality, 8*, 175–89.

Dodge, B., et al. (2012). Beyond "risk": Exploring sexuality among diverse typologies of bisexual men in the United States. *Journal of Bisexuality, 12*, 13–34.

Dolwick-Grieb, S., Davey-Rothwell, M., & Latkin, C. A. (2012). Concurrent partnerships among urban African-American high-risk women with main sex partners. *AIDS & Behavior, 16*, 323–33.

Donham, D. (1998). Freeing South Africa: The modernization of male-male sexuality in Soweto. *Cultural Anthropology, 13*, 3–21.

Dorais, M., & Lajeunesse, S. L. (2004). *Dead Boys Can't Dance: Sexual Orientation, Masculinity, and Suicide*. Montreal: McGill-Queen's University Press.

Dowsett, G. (1996). *Practicing Desire: Homosexual Sex in the Era of AIDS*. Stanford, CA: Stanford University Press.

Dowsett, G. (2002). Sexuality and gender: Diversity and difference. Paper presented at the HIV International AIDS Conference. Barcelona, Spain.

Dowsett, G. W. (2003). Some considerations on sexuality and gender in the context of HIV/AIDS. *Reproductive Health Matters, 11*, 1–9.

Doyal, L. (2002). Putting gender into health and globalization debates: New perspectives and old challenges. *Third World Quarterly, 23*, 233–50.

Doyal, L., Naidoo, J., & Wilton, T. (eds.) (1994). *AIDS: Setting a Feminist Agenda*. London: Taylor & Francis.

Dudgeon, M. S., & Inhorn, M. C. (2004). Men's influences on women's reproductive health: Medical anthropological perspectives. *Social Science & Medicine, 59*, 1379–95.

Dunbar, M. S., Maternowska, M. C., Kang, M. J., Laver, S. M., Mudekunye-Mahaka, I., & Padian, N. S. (2010). Findings from SHAZ! A feasibility study of a microcredit and life-skills HIV prevention intervention to reduce risk among adolescent female orphans in Zimbabwe. *Journal of Prevention and Intervention in the Community, 38*, 147–61.

Dunkle, K. L., & Jewkes, R. K. (2007). Effective HIV prevention requires gender transformative work with men. *Sexually Transmitted Infections, 83*, 173–74.

Dunkle K. L., Jewkes, R. K., Brown, H. C., Gray, G. E., McIntyre, J. A., & Harlow, S. D. (2004). Gender-based violence, relationship power, and risk of HIV infection in women attending antenatal clinics in South Africa. *Lancet, 363*, 1415–21.

Dunkle, K. L., Jewkes, R. K., Nduna, M., Levin, J., Jama, N., Khuzwayo, N., Koss, M. P., & Duvvury, N. (2006). Perpetration of partner violence and HIV risk behaviour among young men in the rural Eastern Cape, South Africa. *AIDS, 20*, 2107–14.

Dunkle, K. L., et al. (2011). Perpetration of violence against women by victims and perpetrators of male-on-male sexual violence in South Africa. Available at http://www.svri.org/forum2011/MaleonMale.pdf

Dupas P., & Robinson, J. (2009). Savings constraints and microenterprise development: Evidence from a field experiment in Kenya. National Bureau of Economic Research, Cambridge, MA. Available at www.econ.ucla.edu/pdupas/savingsconstraints.pdf.

Durant, T., McDavid, K., Hu, X., et al. (2007). Racial/ethnic disparities in diagnoses of HIV/AIDS: 33 states, 2001–2005. *Morbidity and Mortality Weekly Report, 56*, 189–93.

Dworkin, S. L. (2005). Who is epidemiologically fathomable in the HIV/AIDS epidemic? Gender, sexuality, and intersectionality in public health. *Culture, Health, and Sexuality, 7*, 16–23.

Dworkin, S. L. (2010). Masculinity, health, and human rights. *Hastings International Law and Comparative Review, 33*, 461–78.

Dworkin, S. L. (2013). Q&A interview: Changing men in South Africa. *Contexts, Fall*, 8–11.

Dworkin, S. L., & Blankenship, K. (2009). Microfinance: Assessing its promise and limitations. *AIDS & Behavior, 13*, 462–69.

Dworkin, S. L., Colvin, C., Hatcher, A., Peacock, D. (2012). Men's perceptions of women's rights and changing gender relations in South Africa: Lessons for working with men and boys in HIV and anti-violence programs. *Gender & Society, 26*, 97–120.

Dworkin, S. L., Dunbar, M. S., Krishnan, S., Hatcher, A. M., & Sawires, S. (2011). Uncovering tensions and capitalizing on synergies in HIV/AIDS and antiviolence programs. *American Journal of Public Health, 101,* 995–1003.

Dworkin, S. L., & Ehrhardt, A. A. (2007). Going beyond ABC to include GEM (gender relations, economic contexts, and migration movements): Critical reflections on progress in the HIV/AIDS epidemic. *American Journal of Public Health, 97,* 13–16.

Dworkin, S. L., Fullilove, R., & Peacock, D. (2009). Are HIV/AIDS prevention interventions for heterosexually active men gender-specific? A critical look at work in the United States. *American Journal of Public Health, 99,* 981–84.

Dworkin, S. L., Grabe, S., Lu, T., Kwena, Z., Bukusi, E., & Mwaura-Muira, E. (2013). Property rights violations as a structural driver of women's HIV risks in Nyanza and Western Provinces, Kenya. *Archives of Sexual Behavior, 42,* 703–13.

Dworkin, S. L., & Hatcher, A. (2012). Microfinance and health: What works, where, when, why/how? An integrated systematic and critical review of the global evidence base. Prepared for the Centers for Disease Control and Prevention. National Consultation: Economic Intervention Development for Low-Income African-Americans at Risk of HIV/AIDS.

Dworkin, S. L., Hatcher, A., Colvin, C., & Peacock, P. (2013). Impact of a gender-transformative HIV and antiviolence program on gender ideologies and masculinities in two rural, South African communities. *Men and Masculinities, 16,* 181–202.

Dworkin, S. L., & Messner, M. A. (1999). Just do what? Sport, bodies, gender. Pp. 341–64 in J. Lorber, B. Hess, & M. M. Ferree (eds.), *Revisioning Gender.* Thousand Oaks, CA: Sage.

Dworkin, S. L., & O'Sullivan, L. (2005). Actual versus desired initiation patterns: Tapping disjunctures within and departures from traditional male sexual scripts. *Journal of Sex Research, 42,* 150–58.

Dworkin, S. L., & O'Sullivan, L. (2010). "It's less work for us and it shows us she has good taste": Masculinity, sexual initiation, and contemporary sexual scripts. Pp. 105–21 in M. Kimmel (ed.), *The Sexual Self: The Construction of Sexual Scripts.* Nashville, TN: Vanderbilt University Press.

Dworkin, S. L., Swarr, A. L., & Cooky, C. (2013). (In)justice in sport: The treatment of South African track star Caster Semenya. *Feminist Studies, 39,* 40–69.

Dworkin, S. L., Treves-Kagan, S., & Lippman, S. A. (2013). Gender-transformative interventions to reduce HIV risks and violence with heterosexually active men: A review of the global evidence. *AIDS & Behavior, 17,* 2845–63.

Dworkin, S. L., & Wachs, F. L. (2009). *Body Panic: Gender, Health, and the Selling of Fitness.* New York: New York University Press.

Egan, D. (2013). *Becoming Sexual: A Critical Appraisal of the Sexualization of Girls.* Cambridge, UK: Polity.

Ehlers T. B., & Main, K. (1998). Women and the false promise of microenterprise. *Gender & Society, 12,* 424–40.

Ehrhardt, A. A., & Exner, T. M. (2000). Prevention of sexual risk behavior for HIV infection with women. *AIDS, 14,* S53–S58.

Ehrhardt, A. A., Exner, T. M., & Hoffman, S. (2000). HIV/STD risk and sexual strategies among women family planning clients in New York: Project FIO. *AIDS & Behavior, 6,* 1–13.

Ehrhardt, A. A., Exner, T. M., Hoffman, S., et al. (2002). A gender-specific HIV/STD risk reduction intervention for women in a health care setting: Short- and long-term results of a randomized clinical trial. *AIDS Care, 14,* 147–61.

Ehrhardt, A. A., Yingling, S., Zawadski, E., & Martinez-Ramirez, M. (1992). Prevention of heterosexual transmission of HIV: Barriers for women. *Journal of Psychology and Human Sexuality, 5,* 37–67.

Eitzen, D. S., & Baca Zinn, M. B. (1995). Structural transformation and systems of inequality. Pp. 202–6 in M. L. Andersen & P. Hill-Collins (eds.), *Race, Class, and Gender: An Anthology.* Belmont, CA: Wadsworth.

El-Bassel, N., Gilbert, L., Golder, S., et al. (2004). Deconstructing the relationship between intimate partner violence and sexual HIV risk among drug-involved men and their female partners. *AIDS & Behavior, 8,* 429–39.

El-Bassel, N., Witte, S. S., Gilbert, L., Wu, E., Chang, M., Hill, J., et al. (2003). The efficacy of a relationship-based HIV/STD prevention program for heterosexual couples. *American Journal of Public Health, 93,* 963–69.

Elwy, A. R., Hart, G. J., Hawkes, S., & Petticrew, M. (2002). Effectiveness of interventions to prevent sexually transmitted infections and human immunodeficiency virus in heterosexual men: A systematic review. *Archives of Internal Medicine, 162,* 1818–30.

Epprecht, M. (2008). *Heterosexual Africa? The History of an Idea from the Age of Exploration to the Age of AIDS.* Athens: Ohio University Press.

Epprecht, M. (2013). *Sexuality and Social Justice in Africa: Rethinking Homophobia and Forging Resistance.* London: Zed.

Epstein, H. (2008). *The Invisible Cure: Why We Are Losing the Fight against AIDS in Africa.* New York: Picador.

Epstein, S. (1996). A queer encounter: Sociology and the study of sexuality. Pp. 146–67 in Stephen Seidman (ed.), *Queer Theory Sociology.* New York: Wiley-Blackwell.

Exner, T. M., Gardos, P. S., Seal, D. W., & Ehrhardt, A. A. (1999). HIV sexual risk reduction interventions with heterosexual men: The forgotten group. *AIDS and Behavior, 3,* 347–58.

Exner, T. M., Hoffman, S., Dworkin, S., & Ehrhardt, A. A. (2003). Beyond the male condom: The evolution of gender-specific HIV interventions for women. *Annual Review of Sex Research, 14,* 114–36.

Exner, T. M., Seal, D. W., & Ehrhardt, A. A. (1997). A review of HIV interventions for at-risk women. *AIDS & Behavior, 2,* 93–124.

Fausto-Sterling, A. (1985). *Myths of Gender: Biological Theories about Women and Men.* New York: Basic Books.

Fausto-Sterling, A. (2000). *Sexing the Body: Gender Politics and the Construction of Sexuality.* New York: Basic Books.

Featherman, D., Hall, M., & Krislov, M. (eds.) (2009). *The Next 25 Years: Affirmative Action in Higher Education in the United States and South Africa*. Ann Arbor: University of Michigan Press.

Fields, E. L., Fullilove, R. E., & Fullilove, M. (2001). HIV Sexual Risk-taking Behavior among Young Black MSM: Contextual Factors. Atlanta, GA: American Public Health Association Annual Meeting.

Fields, E. L., et al. (2012). HIV risk and perceptions of masculinity among young black men who have sex with men. *Journal of Adolescent Health, 50*, 296–303.

Fischer, H. (2013). Congressional research service report: U.S. military casualty statistics: Operation New Dawn, Operation Iraqi Freedom, and Operation Enduring Freedom. Available at http://www.fas.org/sgp/crs/natsec/RS22452.pdf

Flood, M. (2003a). Lust, trust, and latex: Why young heterosexual men do not use condoms. *Culture, Health, & Sexuality, 5*, 353–69.

Flood, M. (2003b). Addressing the sexual cultures of heterosexual men: Key strategies in involving men and boys in HIV/AIDS prevention. Available at http://www.un.org/womenwatch/daw/egm/men-boys2003/EP6-Flood.pdf

Flood, M. (2007). Involving men in gender practice and policy. *Critical Half, 5*, 9–14.

Flood, M. (2011). Involving men in efforts to end violence against women. *Men & Masculinities, 14*, 358–77. Available at http://www.azrapeprevention.org/sites/azrapeprevention.org/files/Flood.pdf

Flood, M., Peacock, D., Grieg, A., & Barker, G. (2010). Policy approaches to involving men and boys in achieving gender equality and health equity. Geneva, Switzerland: World Health Organization. Available at http://whqlibdoc.who.int/publications/2010/9789241500128_eng.pdf

Ford, C. L., Whetten, K. D., Hall, S. A., Kaufman, J. S., & Thrasher, A. D. (2007). Black sexuality, social construction, and research targeting "the down low" ("the DL"). *Annals of Epidemiology, 17*, 209–16.

Foucault, M. (1978). *The History of Sexuality*. New York: Vintage.

Foucault. M. (1980). *Power/Knowledge: Selected Interviews and Other Writings*. Brighton, UK: Harvester.

Fox-Tierney, R. A., Ickovics, J. R., Cerrata, C., & Ethier, K. A. (1999). Potential sex differences remain understudied: A case study of inclusion of women in HIV/AIDS-related neuropsychological research. *Review of General Psychology, 3*, 44–54.

Freire, P. (1993). *Pedagogy of the Oppressed*. New York: Continuum.

Frenkel, R. (2008). Feminism and contemporary culture in South Africa. *African Studies, 67*, 1–9.

Friedan, B. (1964). *The Feminine Mystique*. New York: Dell.

Friedman, S. (1993). What is the role of structural interventions in HIV prevention? San Francisco: Center for AIDS Prevention Studies. Available at http://caps.ucsf.edu/uploads/pubs/FS/pdf/structuralFS.pdf

Fullilove R. (2006). African Americans, health disparities, and HIV/AIDS: Recommendations for confronting the epidemic in Black America. Available at http://www.nicic.org/Library/022078

Garnett, G. P., & Johnson, A. M. (1997). Coining a new term in epidemiology: Concurrency and HIV. *AIDS, 11,* 681–83.

Gawaya, R., & Mukasa, R. S. (2005). The African women's protocol: A new dimension for women's rights in Africa. *Gender & Development 13,* 42–50.

Gentry, Q. M., Elifson, K., & Sterk, C. (2005). Aiming for more relevant HIV risk reduction: A Black feminist perspective for enhancing HIV prevention for low-income African-American women. *AIDS Education & Prevention, 17,* 238–52.

Gerson, J. M., & Peiss, K. (1985). Boundaries, negotiation, consciousness: Reconceptualising gender relations. Social Problems, 32, 317-31.

Gevisser, M., & Cameron, E. (eds) (1995). *Defiant Desire: Gay and Lesbian Lives in South Africa.* Johannesburg: Ravan.

Global Coalition on Women and AIDS (2006). Economic security for women fights AIDS. Available at http://data.unaids.org/pub/BriefingNote/2006/20060308_BN_GCWA_en.pdf

Glynn, J. R., et al. (2001). Why do young women have a much higher prevalence of HIV than young men? A study in Kisumu, Kenya, and Ndola, Zambia. *Journal of Acquired Immune Deficiency Syndromes, 15,* S51–S60.

Glynn, J. R., et al. (2003). HIV risk in relation to marriage in areas with high prevalence of HIV infection, *Journal of Acquired Immune Deficiency Syndromes, 22,* 526–35.

Goetz, A. M., & Gupta, R. S. (1996). Who takes the credit? Gender, power, and control over loan use in rural credit programs in Bangladesh. *World Development, 24,* 45–64.

Golembeski, C., & Fullilove, R. (2005). Criminal (in)justice in the city and its associated health consequences. *American Journal of Public Health, 95,* 1701–6.

Gollub, E. L. (2000). The female condom: Tool for women's empowerment. *American Journal of Public Health, 90,* 1377–81.

Gómez, C. A., & VanOss Marín, B. (1996). Gender, culture, and power: Barrier to HIV-prevention strategies for women. *Journal of Sex Research, 33,* 355–62.

Grabe, S. (2010). Promoting gender equality: The role of ideology, power, and control in the link between land ownership and violence in Nicaragua. *Analyses of Social Issues and Public Policy, 10,* 146–70.

Grabe, S. (2012). An empirical examination of women's empowerment and transformative change in the context of international development. *American Journal of Community Psychology, 49,* 233–45

Grabe, S., Dutt, A., & Dworkin, S. L. (2014). Women's community mobilization and well-being: Local resistance to global social inequities in Nicaragua and Tanzania. *Journal of Community Psychology, 42,* 379–97.

Greene, M. E., & Biddlecom, A. E. (2000). Absent and problematic men: Demographic accounts of male reproductive roles. *Demography, 26,* 81–115.

Greig, A. (2003). HIV prevention with men: Towards gender equality and social justice. UN Division of Advancement of Women, with ILO, UNAIDS, UNDP. Available at http://www.un.org/womenwatch/daw/egm/men-boys2003/EP7-Greig.pdf

Greig, A., Peacock, D., Msimang, S., & Jewkes, R. (2008). Gender and AIDS: Time to act. *Journal of Acquired Immune Deficiency Syndromes, 22* (S2): S35–S43.

Grieg, F. E., & Koopman, C. (2003). Multilevel analysis of women's empowerment and HIV prevention: Quantitative survey results from a preliminary study in Botswana. *AIDS & Behavior, 7*, 195-208.

Gruskin, L., Gange, S. J., Celentano, D., Schuman, P., Moore, J. S., Zierler, S., & Vlahov, D. (2002). Incidence of violence against HIV-infected and uninfected women: Findings from the HIV epidemiology research (HER) study. *Journal of Urban Health, 79*, 512-24.

Gupta, G. R. (1994). Globalization, women, and the HIV/AIDS epidemic. *Peace Review, 16*, 79-83.

Gupta, G. R. (2001). Gender, sexuality, and HIV/AIDS: The what, the why, and the how. *SIECUS Report, 29*, 6-12.

Gupta, G. R. (2002). Gender Issues in AIDS Research. Paper presented at "Helping Correcting the 10/90 Gap" plenary session on measuring progress in gender issues. Arusha, Tanzania.

Gupta, G. R. (2005). Luncheon remarks on women and AIDS. Available at http://womenandaids.unaids.org/GCWA_SP_Gupta_02Jun05_en.pdf

Gupta, G. R., Parkhurst, J. O., Ogden, J. A., Aggleton, P., & Mahal, A. (2008). Structural approaches to HIV prevention. *Lancet, 372*, 764-75.

Gupta, G. R., & Weiss, E. (1993). Women's lives and sex: Implications for HIV prevention. *Culture and Medical Psychiatry, 17*, 399-412.

Halberstam, J. (2005). *In a Queer Time and Place: Transgender Bodies, Subcultural Lives.* New York: New York University Press.

Hallman, K. (2004). Socioeconomic Disadvantage and Unsafe Sexual Behaviors among Young Women and Men in South Africa. Policy Research Division Working Paper no. 190. New York: Population Council. Available at www.popcouncil.org/uploads/pdfs/wp/190.pdf

Halperin, D. T., & Epstein, H. (2004). Concurrent sexual partnerships help to explain Africa's high HIV prevalence: Implications for prevention. *Lancet, 363*, 4-6.

Hanck, S., West, B., & Tsui, S. (2007). Can microfinance programs reduce HIV risk in developing countries? Policy update. New Haven, CT: Center for Interdisciplinary Research on AIDS, Yale University.

Hankins, C. A., & Handley, M. A. (1992). HIV disease and AIDS in women: Current knowledge and a research agenda. *Journal of Acquired Immune Deficiency Syndromes, 5*, 957-71.

Harawa, N. T., Greenland, S., Bingham, T. A., Johnson, D. F., Cochran, S. D., Cunningham, W. E., et al. (2004). Associations of race/ethnicity with HIV prevalence and HIV-related behaviors among young men who have sex with men in 7 urban centers in the United States. *Journal of Acquired Immune Deficiency Syndrome, 35*, 526-36.

Hardt, M., & Negri, A. (2000). *Empire.* Cambridge, MA: Harvard University Press.

Harrison, A., et al. (2006). Gender role and relationship norms among young adults in South Africa: Measuring the context of masculinity and HIV risk. *Journal of Urban Health, 83*, 709-22.

Harrison, J., Chin, J., & Ficarrotto, T. (1995). Warning: Masculinity may be dangerous to your health. Pp. 235–49 in M. S. Kimmel & M. A. Messner (eds.), *Men's Lives*. Boston: Allyn & Bacon.

Harvey, S. M., & Bird, S. T. (2004). What makes women feel powerful? An exploratory study of relationship power and sexual decision-making for African Americans at risk of HIV. *Women & Health, 39*, 1–18.

Hashemi, S., Schuler, S., & Riley, A. (1996). Rural credit programs and women's empowerment in Bangladesh. *World Development, 23*, 635–53.

Hassim, S. (1999). From presence to power: Women's citizenship in a new democracy. *Agenda, 40*, 35–36.

Hassim, S. (2003). The gender pact and democratic consolidation: Institutionalizing gender equality in the South African state. *Feminist Studies, 29*, 505–28.

Hatcher, A., et al. (2011). Promoting critical consciousness and social mobilization in HIV/AIDS programs: Lessons and curricular tools from a South African intervention. *Health Education Research, 26*, 542–55.

Hays-Mitchell, M. (1999). From survivorship to entrepreneur: Gendered dimensions of microenterprise development in Peru. *Environment and Planning, 31*, 252–72.

Heise, L. (1995). Violence, sexuality, and women's lives. Pp. 109–34 in R. G. Parker & J. H. Gagnon (eds.), *Conceiving Sexuality: Approaches to Sex Research in a Postmodern World*. New York: Routledge.

Herdt, G. (1993). *Ritualized Homosexuality in Melanesia*. Berkeley: University of California Press.

Heywood, L., & Dworkin, S. (2003). *Built to Win: The Female Athlete as Cultural Icon*. Minneapolis: University of Minnesota Press.

Higgins, J. A. (2007). Sexy feminisms and sexual health: Theorizing heterosex, pleasure, and constraint in public health research. *Atlantis, 31*, 72–81.

Higgins J. A., & Hirsch, J. S. (2008). Pleasure and power: Incorporating sexuality and inequality into research on contraceptive use and unintended pregnancy. *American Journal of Public Health, 98*, 1803–13.

Higgins, J. A., Hoffman, S., & Dworkin, S. L. (2010). Rethinking gender, heterosexual men, and women's vulnerability to HIV. *American Journal of Public Health, 100*, 435–45.

Hill-Collins, P. (1986). Learning from the outsider within: The sociological significance of Black feminist thought. *Social Problems, 33*, S14–S32.

Hill-Collins, P. (1990). *Black Feminist Thought: Knowledge, Consciousness, and the Politics of Empowerment*. New York: Routledge.

Hill-Collins, P. (1999). Moving beyond gender: Intersectionality and scientific knowledge. Pp. 261–84 in M. M. Feree, J. Lorber, & B. B. Hess (eds.), *Revisioning Gender*. Thousand Oaks, CA: Sage.

Hill-Collins, P. (2005). *Black Sexual Politics: African-Americans, Gender, and the New Racism*. New York: Routledge.

Hirsch, J. S., Higgins, J., Bentley, M. E., et al. (2002). The social constructions of sexuality: Marital infidelity and sexually transmitted disease; HIV risk in a Mexican community. *American Journal of Public Health, 92*, 1227–37.

Hirsch, J. S., Meneses, S., Thompson, B., Negroni, M., Pelcastre, B., & del Rio, C. (2007). The inevitability of infidelity: Sexual reputation, social geographies, and marital HIV risk in rural Mexico. *American Journal of Public Health, 97*, 986–96.

Hirsch, J. S., Wardlow, H., Smith, D. J., Phinney, H. M., Parikh, S., & Nathanson, C. A. (2010). *The Secret: Love, Marriage, and HIV*. Nashville, TN: Vanderbilt University Press.

Hoad, N. (2005). Introduction. Pp. 14–25 in N. Hoad, K. Martin, & G. Reid (eds.), *Sex & Politics in South Africa*. Cape Town: Double Storey Books.

Hoad, N., Martin, K., & Reid, G. (eds.) (2005). *Sex and Politics in South Africa*. Cape Town: Double Storey Books.

Hobfoll, S. E., Jackson, A. P., & Lavin, J., et al. (2002). Effects and generalizability of communally oriented HIV-AIDS prevention versus general health promotion groups for single, inner-city women in urban clinics. *Journal of Consulting and Clinical Psychology, 70*, 950–60.

Hoffman, S., Exner, T., Mantell, J., & Stein, Z. (2004). The future of the female condom. *Perspectives in Sexual and Reproductive Health, 36*, 120–26.

Holland, J. C., Ramazanoglu, S., Sharpe, S., & Thomson, R. (1994a). Desire, risk, and control: The body as a site of contestation. Pp. 61–80 in L. Doyal, J. Naidoo, & T. Wilton (eds.), *AIDS: Setting a Feminist Agenda*. London: Falmer.

Holland, J. C., Ramazanoglu, S., Sharpe, S., & Thomson, R. (1994b). Achieving masculine sexuality: Young men's strategies for managing vulnerability. Pp. 122–50 in L. Doyal, J. Naidoo, & T. Wilton (eds.), *AIDS: Setting a Feminist Agenda*. London: Falmer.

hooks, b. (1984). *Feminist Theory: From Margin to Center*. Cambridge, MA: South End Press.

hooks, b. (2000). Racism and feminism. Pp. 275–84 in E. Ashton-Jones, Gary A. Olson, & M. Perry (eds.), *The Gender Reader*. Boston: Allyn & Bacon.

Hunter, M. (2004). Masculinities and multiple-sexual-partners in KwaZulu-Natal: The making and unmaking of Isoka. *Transformation, 54*, 123–53.

Hunter, M. (2005). Cultural politics and masculinities: Multiple partners in historical perspective in KwaZulu-Natal. *Culture, Health, & Sexuality, 7*, 209–23.

Hunter, M. (2007). The changing political economy of sex in South Africa: The significance of unemployment and inequalities to the scale of the AIDS pandemic. *Social Science & Medicine, 64*, 689–700.

Hutchinson, S., Weiss, E., Barker, G., Sagundo, M., & Pulerwitz, J. (2004). Involving Young Men in HIV Prevention Programs: Operations Research on Gender-based Approaches in Brazil, Tanzania, and India. Horizons Report, Washington, DC: Population Council; December 2004. Available at http://www.popcouncil.org/horizons/newsletter/horizons(9)_1.html Accessed on March 20, 2008.

International AIDS Alliance (2003). A global conference on reaching men to improve reproductive health for all. Washington, DC. Available at http://www.eldis.org/vfile/upload/1/document/0708/DOC14410.pdf

Isike, C., & Okeke-Uzodike, U. (2008). Modernizing without westernizing: Redefining African patriarchies in the quest to curb HIV and AIDS in Africa. *Journal of Constructive Theology, 14,* 3–20.

Jewkes, R., Dunkle, K., Nduna, M., Levin, J., Jama, N., Khuzwayo, N., et al. (2006). Factors associated with HIV sero-status in young rural South African women: Connections between intimate partner violence and HIV. *International Journal of Epidemiology, 35,* 1461–68.

Jewkes, R., Dunkle, K., Nduna, M., & Shai, N. (2010). Intimate partner violence, relationship power inequity, and incidence of HIV infection in young women in South Africa: A cohort study. *Lancet, 376,* 41–48.

Jewkes, R., Levin, J. B., & Penn-Kekana, L. A. (2003). Gender inequalities, intimate partner violence, and HIV preventive practices: Findings of a South African cross-sectional study. *Social Science & Medicine, 56,* 125–34.

Jewkes, R., & Morrell, R. (2010). Gender and sexuality: Emerging perspectives from the heterosexual epidemic in South Africa and implications for HIV risk and prevention. *Journal of the International AIDS Society, 13.* Available at http://www.ncbi. nlm.nih.gov/pmc/articles/PMC2828994

Jewkes, R., Nduna, M., Levin, J., Jama, N., Khuzwayo, N., Koss, M., Wood, K., Duvvury, N. (2006). A cluster randomized-controlled trial to determine the effectiveness of Stepping Stones in preventing HIV infections and promoting safer sexual behavior amongst youth in the rural Eastern Cape, South Africa: Trial design, methods, and baseline findings. *Tropical Medicine and International Health, 11,* 3–16.

Jewkes, R., Sikweyiya, Y., Morrell, R., & Dunkle, K. (2011). The relationship between intimate partner violence, rape, and HIV amongst South African men: A cross-sectional study. *PLoS ONE, 6,* e24256.

Jordan-Young, R. M. (2010). *Brain Storm: The Flaws in the Science of Sex Differences.* Cambridge, MA: Harvard University Press.

Jurik, N. C. (2005). *Bootstrap Dreams: U.S. Microenterprise Development in an Era of Welfare Reform.* Ithaca, NY: Cornell University Press.

Kabeer, N. (1998). "Money Can't Buy Me Love"? Re-evaluating Gender, Credit, and Empowerment in Rural Bangladesh. Sussex, UK: Institute of Development Studies. Available at https://www.ids.ac.uk/publication/money-can-t-buy-me-love-re-evaluating-gender-credit-and-empowerment-in-rural-bangladesh.

Kahn, J. G., Gurvey, J., Pollack, L. M., Binson, D., & Catania, J. A. (1997). How many HIV infections cross the bisexual bridge? An estimate from the United States. *AIDS, 11,* 1031–37.

Khan, S., Hudson-Rodd, N., Saggers, S., Bhuiyan, M. I., & Bhuiya, A. (2004). Safer sex or pleasurable sex? Rethinking condom use in the AIDS era. Sexual Health, 1, 217–25.

Kaiser Family Foundation (2012a). The global HIV/AIDS epidemic. Available at http://kff.org/global-health-policy/fact-sheet/the-global-hivaids-epidemic

Kaiser Family Foundation (2012b). HIV/AIDS policy fact sheet: The HIV/AIDS epidemic in Washington, DC. Available at http://kaiserfamilyfoundation.files.wordpress.com/2013/01/8335.pdf

Kalichman, S. C. (2010). Social and structural HIV prevention in alcohol-serving establishments: Review of international interventions across populations. *Alcohol Research & Health, 33,* 184–94.

Kalichman, S. C., Cain, D., & Simbayi, L. C. (2011). Multiple recent sexual partnerships and alcohol use among sexually transmitted infection clinic patients, Cape Town, South Africa. *Sexually Transmitted Diseases, 38,* 18–23.

Kalichman, S. C., Roffman, R. A., Picciano, J. F., & Bolan, M. (1998). Risk for HIV infection among bisexual men seeking HIV-prevention services and risks posed to their female partners. *Health Psychology, 17,* 320–27.

Kalichman, S. C., Simbayi, L. C., Cain, D., Cherry, C., Henda, N., & Cloete, A. (2007). Sexual assault, sexual risks, and gender attitudes in a community sample of South African men. *AIDS Care, 19,* 20–27.

Kalichman, S. C., Simbayi, L. C., Cloete, A., Clayford, M., Arnolds, W., Mxoli, M., Smith, G., Cherry, C., Shefer, T., Crawford, M., & Kalichman, M. O. (2009). Integrated gender-based violence and HIV risk reduction for South African men: Results of a quasi-experimental field trial. *Prevention Science, 10,* 260–69.

Kalichman, S. C., Simbayi, L. C., Kaufman, M., Cain, D., & Jooste, S. (2007). Alcohol use and sexual risks for HIV/AIDS in sub-Saharan Africa: Systematic review of empirical findings. *Prevention Science, 8,* 141–51.

Kalichman, S. C., et al. (2008). Randomized trial of a community-based alcohol-related HIV risk reduction intervention for men and women in Cape Town, South Africa. *Annals of Behavioral Medicine, 36,* 270–79.

Kamb, M. L., & Wortley, P. M. (2000). Human immunodeficiency virus and AIDS in women. Pp. 379–89 in M. Goldman & M. Hatch (eds.), *Women and Health.* San Diego: Academic Press.

Kapp, C. (2006). Rape on trial in South Africa. *Lancet, 367,* 718–19.

Karim, N. (2011). *Microfinance and Its Discontents.* Minneapolis: University of Minnesota Press.

Karkazis, K., Jordan-Young, B., Davis, G., & Camporesi, S. (2012). Out of bounds? A critique of the new policies on hyperandrogenism in elite female athletes. *American Journal of Bioethics, 12,* 3–16.

Katz, J. (1995). *The Invention of Heterosexuality.* New York: Penguin.

Kaufman, M. (1994). The construction of masculinity and the triad of men's violence. Pp. 33–55 in L. O'Toole, J. R. Schiffman, & M. K. Edwards (eds.), *Gender Violence: Interdisciplinary Perspectives.* New York: New York University Press.

Kemp, A., et al. (1995). The dawn of a new day: Redefining South African feminisms. In A. Basu (ed.), *The Challenge of Local Feminisms: Women's Movements in Comparative Perspective.* Boulder, CO: Westview.

Kempadoo, K., Sanghera, J., & Patanaik, B. (2011). *Trafficking and Prostitution Reconsidered: New Perspectives on Migration, Sex Work, and Human Rights.* Boulder, CO: Paradigm.

Kerrigan, D., et al. (2006). Environmental-structural interventions to reduce HIV/STI risk among female sex workers in the Dominican Republic. *American Journal of Public Health, 96,* 120–25.

Kim, J., Ferrari, G., Abramsky, T., et al. (2009). Assessing the incremental effects of combining economic and health interventions: The IMAGE study in South Africa. *Bulletin of the World Health Organization, 87,* 824–32.

Kim, J., et al. (2002). Social Interventions for HIV/AIDS Intervention with Microfinance for AIDS and Gender Equity. IMAGE STUDY, RADAR (Rural AIDS and Development Action Research Program) and SEF (Small Enterprise Foundation), Monograph 2: Intervention. Available at www.aidsportal.org/ . . . /Intervention_monograph_no_pics.pdf.pdf

Kim, J. C., & Watts, C. H. (2005). Gaining a foothold: Tackling poverty, gender inequality, and HIV in Africa. *British Medical Journal, 331,* 769–72.

Kim, J. C., Watts, C., Hargreaves, J., et al. (2007). Understanding the impact of a microfinance-based intervention on women's empowerment and the reduction of intimate partner violence. *American Journal of Public Health, 97,* 1794–1802.

Kimmel, M. (1987). Men's responses to feminism at the turn of the century. *Gender & Society, 1,* 261–83.

Kimmel, M. (1990). *Manhood in America: A Cultural History.* New York: Free Press.

Kimmel, M. (1995). Gendering desire. Pp. 3–24 in Michael Kimmel (ed.), *The Gender of Desire.* New York: SUNY Press.

Kimmel, M. (1996). *Manhood in America: A Cultural History.* New York: Free Press.

Kimmel, M. (2000). Saving the males: The sociological implications of the Virginia Military Institute and the Citadel. *Gender & Society, 14,* 494–516.

Kimmel, M., & Mosmiler, M. S. (1992). *Against the Tide: Pro-Feminist Men in the United States, 1776–1990; A Documentary History.* New York: Beacon.

Kinsey, A. C., et al. (1948/1998). *Sexual Behavior in the Human Male.* Philadelphia: W.B. Saunders; Bloomington: Indiana University Press.

Kinsey, A. C., et al. (1953/1998). *Sexual Behavior in the Human Female.* Philadelphia: W.B. Saunders; Bloomington: Indiana University Press.

Kippax, S., Stephenson, N., Parker, R., & Aggleton, P. (2013). Between individual agency and structure in HIV prevention: Understanding the middle ground of social practice. *American Journal of Public Health, 103,* 1367–75.

Klein, A. (1993). *Little Big Men: Bodybuilding Subculture and Gender Construction.* New York: SUNY Press.

Klein, A. (1995). Life's too short to die small. Pp. 105–20 in D. Sabo & D. F. Gordon (eds.), *Men's Health and Illness: Gender, Power, and the Body.* New York: Sage.

Klein, F. (1999). *The Bisexual Option.* New York: Routledge.

Kline, A., Kline, E., & Oken, E. (1992). Minority women and sexual choice in the age of AIDS. *Social Science & Medicine, 34,* 447–57

Kmietowicz, Z. (2004). Women are being let down in efforts to stem HIV/AIDS. *British Medical Journal, 328,* 305.

Knight, R. H. (1994). How domestic partnerships and gay marriage threaten the family. In R. M. Baird and S. E. Rosenbaum (eds.) (2004). *Same-Sex Marriage: The Moral and Legal Debate.* New York: Prometheus Books.

Krishnan, S., Dunbar, M. S., Minnis, A. M., Medlin, C. A., Gerdts, C. E., & Padian, N. S. (2008). Poverty, gender inequities, and women's risk of human immunodeficiency virus/AIDS. *Annals of the New York Academy of Science, 1136,* 101–10.

Krishnan, S., Rocca, C., Hubbard, A. E., Subbiah, K., Edmeades, J., & Padian, N. S. (2010). Do changes in spousal employment status lead to domestic violence? Insights from a prospective study in Bangalore, India. *Social Science & Medicine, 70,* 136–43.

Kynoch, G. (2005). Crime, conflict, and politics in transition-era South Africa. *African Affairs, 104,* 493–514.

Laing, A. (2012). South Africa's whites still paid six times more than blacks. *Telegraph,* October 30, 2012. Available online.

Landau, L. B., & Misago, J. B. (2009). Who's to blame and what's to gain: Reflections on space, states, and violence in Kenya and South Africa. *Africa Spectrum, 44,* 99–110.

Lang, D. L., Salazar, L. F., DiClemente, R. J., & Markosyan, K. (2013). Gender-based violence as a risk factor for HIV-associated risk behaviors among sex workers in Armenia. *AIDS & Behavior, 17,* 551–58.

Lang, S. (1999). Lesbians, men-women, and two-spirits: Homosexuality and gender in Native American cultures. Pp. 91–118 in E. Blackwood & S. E. Wieringa (eds.), *Same-Sex Relations and Female Desires: Transgender Practices across Cultures.* New York: Columbia University Press.

Langlands, R. (2006). *Sexual Morality in Ancient Rome.* Cambridge: Cambridge University Press.

Laqueur, T. (1990). *Making Sex: Body and Gender from the Greeks to Freud.* Cambridge, MA: Harvard University Press.

Larance, L. Y. (1998). Building social capital from the centre: A village-level investigation of Bangladeshís Grameen Bank. Center for Social Development Working Paper. 98–94. Available at http://www.microfinancegateway.org/library/building-social-capital-centre-village-level-investigation-bangladeshs-grameen-bank

Lemke, T. (2011). *Biopolitics: An Introduction.* New York: New York University Press.

Lerum, K. (1999). 12-Step feminism makes sex workers sick: How the state and the recovery movement turn radical women into "Useless Citizens." *Sexuality & Culture, 2,* 7–36.

Logan, T. K., Cole, J., & Leukefeld, C. (2002). Women, sex, and HIV: Social and contextual factors, meta-analysis of published interventions, and implications for practice and research. *Psychological Bulletin, 128,* 851–85.

Lorber, J. (1994). *Paradoxes of Gender.* New Haven, CT: Yale University Press.

Lorber, J. (1996). Beyond the binaries: Depolarizing the categories of sex, sexuality, and gender. *Sociological Inquiry, 66,* 143–59.

Lorber, J. (1999). Embattled terrain: Gender and sexuality. In M. Feree, J. Lorber, & B. Hess (eds.), *Revisioning Gender.* Thousand Oaks, CA: Sage.

Lorde, A. (2007). *Sister Outsider: Essays and Speeches by Audre Lorde.* New York: Random House.

Loren, L. B., & Misago, J. B. (2009). Who's to blame and what's to gain: Reflections on space, state, and violence in Kenya and South Africa. *Africa Spectrum, 44*, 99–110.

Lotfi, R., Tehrani, F. R., Khoei, E. M., Yaghmaei, F., & Dworkin, S. L. (2013). How do women at risk of HIV/AIDS in Iran perceive gender norms and gendered power relations in the context of safer sex negotiations? *Archives of Sexual Behavior, 42*, 873–81.

Lozano, R., Naghavi, M., Foreman, K., et al. (2012). Global and regional mortality from 235 causes of death for 20 age groups in 1990 and 2010: A systematic analysis for the Global Burden of Disease Study 2010. *Lancet, 380*, 2095–2128.

Lu, T., Kwena, Z., Zwicker, L., Bukusi, E., Maura-Muira, E., & Dworkin, S. (2013). Securing women's property rights in the era of HIV/AIDS: Barriers and facilitators of implementing a community-led structural intervention in Western Kenya. *AIDS Education and Prevention, 25*, 151–63.

Luke, N. (2003). Age and economic asymmetries in the sexual relationships of adolescent girls in sub-Saharan Africa. *Studies in Family Planning, 34*, 67–86.

Lupton, D. (1995). *The Imperative of Health: Public Health and the Regulated Body.* London: Sage.

Lurie, M. (2000). Migration and AIDS in southern Africa: A review. *South African Journal of Science, 96*, 343–47.

Lurie, M. N., Williams, B. G., Zuma, K., Mkaya-Mwamburi, D., Garnett, G. P., Sturm, A. W., et al. (2003). The impact of migration on HIV-1 transmission in South Africa: A study of migrant and nonmigrant men and their partners. *Sexually Transmitted Diseases 30*, 149–56.

Lurie, M. N., Williams, B. G., Zuma, K., Mkaya-Mwamburi, D., Garnett, G. P., Sweat, M. D., et al. (2003). Who infects women? HIV-1 concordance and discordance among migrant and non-migrant couples in South Africa. *AIDS, 17*, 2245–52.

Luyt, R. (2003). Rhetorical representations of masculinities in South Africa: Moving towards a material discursive understanding of men. *Journal of Community & Applied Social Psychology, 13*, 46–69.

Luyt, R. (2012). Representations of masculinities and race in South African television advertising. *Journal of Gender Studies, 21*, 35–60.

Lyles, C., Kay, L. S., Crepaz, N., Herbst, J. H., Passin, W. F., et al. (2007). Best-evidence interventions: Findings from a systematic review of HIV behavioral interventions for US populations at high risk, 2000–2004. *American Journal of Public Health, 97*, 133–43.

Maartens, G., Wood, R., O'Keefe, E., & Byrne, C. (1997). Independent epidemics of heterosexual and homosexual HIV infection in South Africa. *QJM: An International Journal of Medicine, 90*, 449–54.

Machtinger, E. L., Haberer, J. E., Wilson, T. C., & Weiss, D. S. (2012a). Psychological trauma and PTSD in HIV-positive women: A meta-analysis. *AIDS & Behavior, 16*, 2091–2100.

Machtinger, E. L. Haberer, J. E., Wilson, T. C., & Weiss, D. S. (2012b). Recent trauma is associated with antiretroviral failure and HIV transmission risk behavior among HIV-positive women and female-identified transgenders. *AIDS & Behavior, 16*, 2160–70.

Mackenzie, S. (2013). *Structural Intimacies: Sexual Stories in the Black AIDS Epidemic.* New Brunswick. NJ: Rutgers University Press.

MacPhail, C., Williams, B. G., & Campbell, C. (2002). Relative risk of HIV infection among young men and women in a South African township. *International Journal of STD and AIDS, 13*, 331–42.

Mahay, J., Laumann, E. O., & Michaels, S. (2001). Race, gender, and class in sexual scripts. Pp. 197–238 in E. O. Laumann & R. T. Michael (eds.), *Sex, Love, and Health in America: Private Choices and Public Policies.* Chicago: University of Chicago Press.

Mahmud, S. (2003). Actually how empowering is microcredit? *Development and Change, 34*, 577–605.

Majors, R., & Billson, J. M. (1992). *Cool Pose: The Dilemmas of Black Manhood in America.* New York: Lexington Books.

Malebranche, D. J. (2008). Bisexually active Black men in the United States and HIV: Acknowledging more than the "down low." *Archives of Sexual Behavior, 37*, 810–16.

Malebranche, D. J., Arriola, K. J., Jenkins, T. R., Dauria, E., & Patel, S. M. (2010). Exploring the "Bisexual Bridge": A qualitative study of risk behavior and disclosure of same-sex behavior among black bisexual men. *American Journal of Public Health, 100*, 159–64.

Malebranche, D. J., Fields, E. L., Bryant, L. O., et al. (2009). Masculine socialization and sexual risk behaviors among Black men who have sex with men. *Men & Masculinities, 12*, 90–112.

Maman, S., Mbwambo, J. K., Hogan, N. M., Kilonzo, G. P., Campbell, J. D., Weiss, E., et al. (2002). HIV-positive women report more lifetime partner violence: Findings from a voluntary counselling and testing clinic in Dar es Salaam, Tanzania. *American Journal of Public Health, 92*, 1331–37.

Manopaiboon, C., Bunnell, R. E., & Kilmarx, P. H., et al. (2003). Leaving sex work: Barriers, facilitating factors, and consequences for female sex workers in northern Thailand. *AIDS Care, 15*, 39–52.

Mantell, J., Dworkin, S. L., Exner, T. M., Hoffman, S., Smit, J. A., & Susser, I. (2006). The promises and limits of female-initiated methods of HIV/STI protection. *Social Science & Medicine, 63*, 1998–2009.

Marais, H. (1998). *South Africa: Limits to Change; The Political Economy of Transition.* New York: Palgrave.

Marais, H. (2005). *Buckling: The Impact of HIV in South Africa.* Center for the Study of AIDS. Pretoria, South Africa. Available at http://www.sarpn.org/documents/d0001789/Buckling_AIDS_2005_Full.pdf

Marks, S. (2002). An epidemic waiting to happen. *African Studies, 61*, 13–26.

Maulsby, C., et al. (2013). HIV among black men who have sex with men in the United States: A review of the literature. *AIDS & Behavior, 18*, 10–25.

Maxwell, C., & Boyle, M. (1995). Risky heterosexual practices amongst women over 30: Gender, power, and long-term relationships. *AIDS Care, 7*, 277–93.

Mayoux, L. (1998). Women's empowerment and micro-finance programmes: Strategies for increasing impact. *Development in Practice, 8*, 235–41.

Mayoux, L. (2001). Women's empowerment versus sustainability? Towards a new paradigm in micro-finance programmes. Pp. 245–70 in B. Lemire, R. Pearson, & G. Campbell (eds.), *Women and Credit: Researching the Past, Refiguring the Future.* New York: Berg.

Mayoux, L. (2005). Women's empowerment through sustainable microfinance: Rethinking "best practice." Available at http://www.sed.manchester.ac.uk/research/iarc/ediais/pdf/WomensEmpowermentthroughSustainableMicrofinance.pdf

Mays, V. M., Cochran, S. D., & Zamudio, A. (2004). HIV prevention research: Are we meeting the need of African American men who have sex with men? *Journal of Black Psychology, 30,* 78–103.

McKay, J. (1997). *Managing Gender: Affirmative Action and Organizational Power in Australian, Canadian, and New Zealand Sport.* New York: SUNY Press.

McNair, L., & Prather, C. (2004). African American women and AIDS: Factors influencing risk and reaction to HIV disease. *Journal of Black Psychology, 30,* 106–23.

Medical Research Council (MRC) (2009). South African national HIV prevalence, incidence, behavior, & communication survey, 2008. Available at http://www.mrc.ac.za/pressreleases/2009/sanat.pdf

Meer, S. (2005). Freedom for women: Mainstreaming gender in the South African liberation struggle and beyond. *Gender & Development, July,* 36–45.

Messner, M. A. (1990). *Power at Play: Sports and the Problem of Masculinity.* Boston: Beacon.

Messner, M. A. (1997). *The Politics of Masculinities: Men in Movements.* Thousand Oaks, CA: Sage.

Messner, M. A. (2002). *Taking the Field: Women, Men, and Sports.* Minneapolis: University of Minnesota Press.

Messner, M. A., & Stevens, M. A. (2002). Scoring without consent: Confronting male athletes' violence against women. Pp. 225–41 in Gatz, M., Messner, M. A., & Ball-Rokeach, S. J. (eds.), *Paradoxes of Youth and Sport.* New York: SUNY Press.

Meyer, I. (2003). Prejudice, social stress, and mental health in gay, lesbian, and bisexual populations: Conceptual issues and research evidence. *Psychological Bulletin, 129,* 674–97.

Miller, S., et al. (2000). A gender-specific intervention for at-risk women. *AIDS Care, 12,* 603–12.

Millett, G., Malebranche, D., Mason, B., & Spikes, P. (2005). Focusing "down low": Bisexual black men, HIV risk, and heterosexual transmission. *Journal of the National Medical Association, 97,* 52–59.

Millett, G. A., Flores, S. A., Peterson, J. L., & Bakeman, R. (2007). Explaining disparities in HIV infection among black and white men who have sex with men: A meta-analysis of HIV risk behaviors. *AIDS, 15,* 2083–91.

Millett, G. A., Peterson, J. L., Wolitski, R. J., & Stall, R. (2006). Greater risk for HIV infection of black men who have sex with men: A critical literature review. *American Journal of Public Health, 96,* 1007–19.

Mishra, V., Assche, S. B., Greener, R., Vaessen, M., Hong, R., Ghys, P. D., et al. (2007). HIV infection does not disproportionately affect the poorer in sub-Saharan Africa. *AIDS, 21,* S17–28.

MMWR (2011). Increase in newly diagnosed HIV infections among Black MSM— Milwaukee County, Wisconsin, 1999–2008. Available at http://www.cdc.gov/mmwr/ preview/mmwrhtml/mm6004a3.htm

Moffett, H. (2008). Gender. Pp. 104–14 in N. Shepherd & S. Robins (eds.), *New South African Keywords.* Johannesburg: Jacana Media.

Montgomery, C. M., V. Hosegood, J. Busza, & I. M. Timaeus (2006). Men's involvement in the South African family: Engendering change in the AIDS era. *Social Science & Medicine, 62,* 2411–19.

Montgomery, J. P., Mokotoff, E. D., Gentry, A. C., & Blair, J. M. (2003). The extent of bisexual behavior in HIV-infected men and implications for transmission to their female sex partners. *AIDS Care, 15,* 829–37.

Moodie, T. D., Ndatshe, V., & Sibuyi, B. (1988). Migrancy and male sexuality on the South African gold mines. *Journal of Southern Africa Studies, 14,* 228–56.

Morduch, J. (1999). The microfinance promise. *Journal of Economic Literature, 37,* 1569–1614. Available at http://www.nyu.edu/projects/morduch/documents/microfinance/Microfinance_Promise.pdf

Morduch, J. (2000). The microfinance schism. *World Development, 28,* 617–29.

Morojele, M. K., et al. (2006). Alcohol use and sexual behavior among risky drinkers and bar and shebeen patrons in Gauteng Province, South Africa. *Social Science & Medicine, 62,* 217–27.

Morrell, R. (1998). Of boys and men: Masculinity and gender in Southern African studies. *Journal of Southern African Studies, 24,* 605–30.

Morrell, R. (ed.) (2001). *Changing Men in Southern Africa.* London: Zed.

Morrell, R. (2002). Men, movements, & gender transformation in South Africa. *Journal of Men's Studies, 10,* 309–27.

Morrell, R., & Jewkes, R. (2011). Carework and caring: A path to gender-equitable practices among men in South Africa? *International Journal of Equity in Health, 10,* 10–17.

Morrell, R., Jewkes, R., & Lindegger, G. (2012). Hegemonic masculinity/masculinities in South Africa: Culture, power, and gender politics. *Men & Masculinities, 15,* 11–30.

Morrell, R., Jewkes, R., Lindegger, G., & Hamlall, V. (2013). Hegemonic masculinity: Reviewing the gendered analysis of men's power in South Africa. *South African Review of Sociology, 44,* 3–21.

Morrell, R., Posel, D. R., & Devey, R. M. (2003). Counting fathers in South Africa: Issues of definition, methodology, and policy. *Social Dynamics, 29,* 73–94.

Morris M., & Kretzschmar, M. (1997). Concurrent partnerships and the spread of HIV. *AIDS, 11,* 641–48.

Morrow, K. M., & Allsworth, J. E. (2000). Sexual risk in lesbians and bisexual women. *Journal of the Gay and Lesbian Medical Association, 4,* 159–65.

Mubangizi, J. C. (2012). A South African perspective on the clash between culture and human rights, with particular reference to gender-related cultural practices and traditions. *Journal of International Women's Studies, 13*, 33–48.

Muñoz-Laboy, M. A., & Dodge, B. (2005). Bisexual practices: Patterns, meanings, and implications for HIV/STI prevention among bisexually active Latino men and their partners. *Journal of Bisexuality, 5*, 81–100.

Munro, B. (2012). *South Africa and the Dream of Love to Come: Queer Sexuality and the Struggle for Freedom*. Minneapolis: University of Minnesota Press.

Mutchler, M., Bogart, L. M., et al. (2008). Psychosocial correlates of unprotected sex without disclosure of HIV positivity among African-American, White, and Latino men who have sex with men and women. *Archives of Sexual Behavior, 37*, 736–47.

Naidoo, V., & Kongolo, M. (2004). Has affirmative action reached South African women? *Journal of International Women's Studies, 6*, 124–36.

Namaste, K. (1994). The politics of inside/out: Queer theory, poststructuralism, and a sociological approach to sexuality. *Sociological Theory, 12*, 220–31.

Newsome, V., & Airhihenbuwa, C. O. (2013). Gender ratio imbalance effects on HIV risk behaviors in African American women. *Health Promotion Practice, 14*, 459–63.

Nguyen, V. K. (2005). Antiretroviral globalism, biopolitics, and therapeutic citizenship. Pp. 124–44 in A. Ong & S. J. Collier (eds.), *Global Assemblages: Technology, Politics, and Ethics as Anthropological Problems*. Oxford: Blackwell.

Niehaus, I. (2009). Renegotiating masculinity in the lowveld: Narratives of male-male sex in compounds, prisons, and at home. Pp. 85–111 in M. Steyn & M. van Zyl (eds.), *The Prize and the Price: Shaping Sexualities in South Africa*. Cape Town: HSRC Press.

Nnko, S., Boerma, J. T., Urassa, M., Mwaluko, G., & Zaba, B. (2004). Secretive females or swaggering males? An assessment of the quality of sexual partnership reporting in rural Tanzania. *Social Science & Medicine, 59*, 299–310.

Nunn, A., et al. (2012). Concurrent sexual partnerships among African American women in Philadelphia: Results from a qualitative study. *Sexual Health, 9*, 288–96.

Obermeyer, C. M. (2006). HIV in the Middle East, *BMJ, 333*, 21.

Office of National AIDS Strategy (2010). National AIDS strategy for the United States. Available at http://aids.gov/federal-resources/national-hiv-aids-strategy/nhas.pdf

O'Leary, A. (2002). Women at risk for HIV from a primary partner: Balancing risk and intimacy. *Annual Review of Sex Research, 11*, 191–234.

Ortiz-Torres, B., Williams, S. P., & Ehrhardt, A. A. (2003). Urban women's gender scripts: Implications for HIV. *Culture, Health, & Sexuality, 5*, 1–17.

O'Sullivan, L. F., & Byers, E. S. (1992). College students' incorporation of initiator and restrictor roles in sexual dating interactions. *Journal of Sex Research, 29*, 435–46.

O'Toole, L. L., Schiffman, J., & Kiter-Edwards, M. L. (eds.). (2007). *Gender Violence: Interdisciplinary Perspectives*. New York: New York University Press.

Padian, N., Shiboski, S., Glass, S., Vittinghoff, E. (1997). Heterosexual transmission of human immunodeficiency virus in northern California: Results from a ten-year study. *American Journal of Epidemiology, 146*, 350–57.

Paiva, V. (2002). Gendered sexual scripts and the sexual scene: Promoting sexual subjects among Brazilian teenagers. In R. Parker, R. Barbosa, & P. Aggleton (eds.), *Framing the Sexual Subject: The Politics of Gender, Sexuality, and Power*. Berkeley: University of California Press.

Parker, R. (1999a). "Within four walls": Brazilian sexual culture and HIV/AIDS. Pp. 253–66 in R. Parker & P. Aggleton (eds.), *Culture, Society, and Sexuality: A Reader*. Philadelphia: Taylor & Francis.

Parker, R. (1999b). *Beneath the Equator: Cultures of Desire, Male Homosexuality, and Emerging Gay Communities in Brazil*. New York: Routledge.

Parker, R., Easton, D., & Klein, C. H. (2000). Structural barriers and facilitators in HIV prevention: A review of international research. *AIDS, 14*, S22–S32.

Parsons, T., & Bales, R. F. (1955). *Family, Socialization, & Interaction Process*. New York: Free Press.

Pascoe, C. J. (2011). *Dude, You're a Fag: Masculinity and Sexuality in High School*. Berkeley: University of California Press.

Patton, C. (1990). *Inventing AIDS*. New York: Routledge.

Patton, C. (2002). *Globalizing AIDS*. Minneapolis: University of Minnesota Press.

Peacock, D. (2002). The Men as Partners Program: Working with Men in South Africa to End Violence against Women and Prevent HIV/AIDS. Engender Health document distributed at XIV International HIV/AIDS Conference Held in Barcelona, Spain.

Peacock, D. (2003). Men as partners: Promoting men's involvement in care and support activities for people living with HIV and AIDS. Available at https://www.un.org/womenwatch/daw/egm/men-boys2003/EP5-Peacock.pdf

Peacock, D. (2013). South Africa's Sonke Gender Justice Network: Educating men for gender equality. *AGENDA: Empowering women for gender equity*. DOI:10.1080/1013 0950.2013.808793. Available online.

Peacock, D., Khumalo, B., & McNab, E. (2006). Men and gender activism in South Africa: Observations, critique, and recommendations for the future. *Agenda, 69*, 76–82.

Peacock, D., & Levack, A. (2004). The men as partners program in South Africa: Reaching men to end gender-based violence and promote sexual and reproductive health. *International Journal of Men's Health, 3*, 173–88.

Peacock, D., Stemple, L., Sawires, S., & Coates, T. J. (2009). Men, HIV/AIDS, and human rights. *Journal of Acquired Immune Deficiency Syndromes, 51*, S119–25.

Pearson, R. (2001). Micro-credit as a path from welfare to work: The experience of the Full Circle Project, UK. Pp. 167–77 in B. Lemire, R. Pearson, & G. Grace Campbell (eds.), *Women and Credit: Researching the Past, Refiguring the Future*. Oxford: Berg.

Petersen, A., & Lupton, D. (1996). *The New Public Health: Health and Self in the Age of Risk*. London: Sage.

Peterson, J. L., & Jones, K. T. (2009). HIV prevention for black men who have sex with men in the United States. *American Journal of Public Health, 99*, 976–80.

Petryna, A. (2002). *Life Exposed: Biological Citizens after Chernobyl*. Princeton, NJ: Princeton University Press.

Pfeiffer, J., & Chapman, R. (2010). Anthropological perspectives on structural adjustment and public health. *Annual Review of Anthropology, 39*, 149–65.

Phetla, G., Busza, J., Hargreaves, J. R., et al. (2008). They have opened our mouths: Increasing women's skills and motivation for sexual communication with young people in rural South Africa. *AIDS Education & Prevention, 20*, 504–18.

Pile, J. M., Bumin, C., Ciloglu, G. A., & Akin, A. (1999). Involving men as partners in reproductive health: Lessons learned from Turkey. AVSC Working Paper #12. Engenderhealth. Available at www.engenderhealth.org

Pleck, J. H. (1981). *The Myth of Masculinity*. Cambridge, MA: MIT Press.

Pleck, J. H. (1983). The theory of male sex role identity: Its rise and fall, 1936–present. Pp. 205–25 in M. Lewin (ed.), *In the Shadow of the Past: Psychology Portrays the Sexes*. New York: Columbia University Press.

Pleck, J. H., Sonenstein, F., & Ku, L. (1993). Masculinity ideology: Its impact on adolescent males' heterosexual relationships. *Journal of Social Issues, 49*, 11–29.

Plummer, K. (2000). Sexualities in a Runaway World: Utopian and Dystopian Challenges. Paper presented at Ford Foundation Workshop on Sexuality and Social Change: An Agenda for Research and Action in the 21st Century, Rio de Janeiro.

Pool, R., Hart, G. J., Green, G., Harrison, S., Nyanzi, S., & Whitworth, J. A. G. (2000). Men's attitudes to condoms and female-controlled means of protection against HIV and STDs in southwestern Uganda. *Culture, Health, & Sexuality, 2*, 197–211.

Population Council (2006). Yaari Dosti: Young men redefine masculinity. New Delhi. Available at www.popcouncil.org/pdfs/yaaridostiend.pdf

Posel, D. (2004). Afterword: Vigilantism and the burden of rights; reflections on the paradoxes of freedom in post-apartheid South Africa. *African Studies, 62*, 231–36.

Posel, D. (2008). AIDS. Pp. 13–24 in N. Shepherd & S. Robins (eds.), *New South African Keywords*. Athens: Ohio University Press.

Preston-Whyte, E., Varga, C., Oosthuizen, H., Roberts, R., & Blose, F. (2000). Survival sex and HIV/AIDS in an African city. Pp. 165–90 in R. Parker, R. M. Barbosa, & P. Aggleton (eds.), *Framing the Sexual Subject: The Politics of Gender, Sexuality, and Power*. Berkeley: University of California Press.

Pronyk, P. M., Hargreaves, J. R., Kim, K., Morison, L. A., Phetla, F., Watts, C., et al. (2006). Effect of a structural intervention for the prevention of intimate partner violence and HIV in rural South Africa: Results of a cluster randomized trial. *Lancet, 368*, 1973–83.

Pronyk, P. M., Kim, J. C., Abramsky, T., Phetla, G., Hargreaves, J. R., Morison, L. A., & Porter, J. D. (2008). A combined microfinance and training intervention can reduce HIV risk behaviour in young female participants. *AIDS, 22*, 1659–65.

Pronyk, P. M., Kim, J. C., Hargreaves, J. R., Makhubele, M. B., Morison, L. A., Watts, C. H., et al. (2005). Microfinance and HIV prevention: Perspectives and emerging lessons from rural South Africa. *Small Enterprise Development, 16*, 26–38.

Pulerwitz, J., Amaro, H., DeJong, W., Gortmaker, S. L., & Rudd, R. (2002). Relationship power, condom use, and HIV risk among women in the USA. *AIDS Care, 14*, 789–800.

Pulerwitz, J., & Barker, G. (2008). Measuring attitudes towards gender norms in Brazil: Development and psychometric evaluation of the GEM scale. *Men & Masculinities, 10*, 322–38.

Pulerwitz, J., & Dworkin, S. L. (2006). "Give and take" in safer sex negotiations: The fluidity of gender-based power relations. *Sexuality Research and Social Policy, 3*, 40–51.

Pulerwitz, J., Gortmaker, S. L., & DeJong, W. (2000). Measuring sexual relationship power in HIV/STD research. *Sex Roles, 42*, 637–60.

Pulerwitz, J., Martin, S., Mehta, M., Castillo, T., Kidanu, A., Verani, F., & Tewolde, S. (2010). *Promoting Gender Equity for HIV and Violence Prevention: Results from the Male Norms Initiative Evaluation in Ethiopia.* Washington, DC: PATH. Available online.

Pulerwitz, J., Michaelis, A., Verma, R., & Weiss E. (2010). Addressing gender dynamics and engaging men in HIV programs: Lessons learned from Horizon research. *Public Health Reports, 125*, 282–92.

Rahman, A. (1999). *Women and Microcredit in Rural Bangladesh: Anthropological Study of the Rhetoric and Realities of Grameen Bank Lending:* Boulder, CO: Westview.

Raj, A., & Bowleg, L. (2012). Heterosexual risk of HIV among Black men in the United States: A call to action against a neglected crisis in Black communities. *American Journal of Men's Health, 6*, 178–81.

Raj, A., Dasgupta, A., Goldson, I., Lafontant, D., Freeman, E., & Silverman, J. G. (2013). Pilot evaluation of the Making Employment Needs [MEN] Count intervention: Addressing behavioral and structural HIV risks in heterosexual Black men. *AIDS Care,* Epub 2013/06/19. PubMed PMID: 23767788.

Ramjee, G., & Gouws, E. (2002). Prevalence of HIV among truck drivers visiting sex workers in KwaZulu-Natal, South Africa. *Sexually Transmitted Diseases, 29*, 44–49.

Ramphele, M., & Richter, L. (2006). Migrancy, family dissolution, and fatherhood. Pp. 73–81 in L. Richter & R. Morrell (eds.), *Baba: Men and Fatherhood in South Africa.* Cape Town: HSRC Press.

Rankin, K. N. (2002). Social capital, microfinance, and the politics of development. *Journal of Feminist Economics, 8*, 1–24.

Ratele, K. (2009). Apartheid, anti-apartheid, and post-apartheid sexualities. Pp. 290–305 in M. Steyn & M. van Zyl (eds.), *The Prize and the Price: Shaping Sexualities in South Africa.* Cape Town: HSRC Press.

Raymond, H. F., & McFarland, W. (2009). Racial mixing and HIV risk among men who have sex with men. *AIDS & Behavior, 13*, 630–37.

Reddy, V., & Sandfort, T. (2011). Researching MSM in South Africa: Some preliminary notes from the front lines in a hidden epidemic. *Feminist Africa, 11*, 29–52. Available at http://agi.ac.za/sites/agi.ac.za/files/fa_11_5_feature_article_2.pdf

Reddy, V., Sandfort, T., & Rispel, L. (eds.) (2010). *From Social Silence to Social Science: Same-Sex Sexuality, HIV & AIDS, and Gender in South Africa.* Cape Town: HSRC Press.

Reeves, T. (2003). Female to female transmission: Seeking answers and challenging myths. *HIV Australia, 2*, 29–30.

Reid, P. T. (2000). Women, ethnicity, and AIDS: What's love got to do with it? *Sex Roles, 42*, 709–22.

Rhodes, S. D., McCoy, T. P., & Vissman, A. T., et al. (2011). A randomized controlled trial of a culturally congruent intervention to increase condom use and HIV testing among heterosexually active immigrant Latino men. *AIDS & Behavior, 15*, 1764–75.

Rich, A. (1982). Compulsory heterosexuality and lesbian existence. Pp. 227–53 in H. Abelove, M. A. Barale, & D. M. Halperin (eds.), *The Lesbian and Gay Studies Reader*. New York: Routledge.

Richardson, D. (1996). Heterosexuality and social theory. Pp. 1–20 in D. Richardson (ed.), *Theorizing Heterosexuality*. Buckingham, UK: Open University Press.

Richter, L., & Morrell, R. (eds.) (2006). *Baba: Men and Fatherhood in South Africa*. Cape Town: HSRC Press.

Riley, E., et al. (2007). Poverty, unstable housing, and HIV infection among women living in the United States. *Current HIV/AIDS Reports, 4*, 1548–68.

Rivers, K., & Aggleton, P. (1999). Men and the HIV epidemic, gender and the HIV epidemic. New York: United Nations Development Programme, HIV and Development Program. Available at http://www.undp.org/content/dam/aplaws/publication/en/publications/hiv-aids/men-and-the-hiv-epidemic/85.pdf

Robins, S. (2008a). *From Revolution to Rights in South Africa: Social Movements, NGOs, and Popular Politics after Apartheid*. Scottsville, South Africa: University of Kwa-Zulu Natal Press.

Robins, S. (2008b). Rights. Pp. 182–94 in N. Shepherd & S. Robins (eds.), *New South African Keywords*. Athens: Ohio University Press.

Rodriguez-Rust, P. (1999). *Bisexuality in the United States*. New York: Columbia University Press.

Rose, N., & Novas, C. (2005). Biological citizenship. In A. Ong & S. J. Collier (eds.), *Global Assemblages, Technology, and Ethics as Anthropological Problems*. Oxford: Blackwell.

Ross, M. W., Essien, E. J., Williams, M. L., & Fernandez-Esquer, M. E. (2003). Concordance between sexual behavior and sexual identity in street outreach samples of four racial/ethnic groups. *Sexually Transmitted Diseases, 30*, 110–13.

Roy, A. (2010). *Poverty Capital: Microfinance and the Making of Development*. New York: Routledge.

Royce, R. A., Sena, A., Cates, W., & Cohen, M. S. (1997). Sexual transmission of HIV. *New England Journal of Medicine, 336*, 1072–78.

Rubin, G. (1975). The traffic in women: Notes on the political economy of sex. In R. Reiter (ed.), *Towards an Anthropology of Women*. New York: Monthly Review Press.

Rubin, G. (1999). Thinking sex: Notes for a radical theory of the politics of sexuality. Pp. 143–78 in R. Parker & P. Aggleton (eds.), *Culture, Society, and Sexuality: A Reader*. Philadelphia: Taylor & Francis.

Rutter, V., & Schwartz, P. (2011). *The Gender of Sexuality*. Lanham, MD: Rowman & Littleton.

Sabo, D., & Gordon, F. (1995). Rethinking men's health and illness. Pp. 1–21 in D. Sabo & D. F. Gordon (eds.), *Men's Health and Illness, Gender, Power, and the Body*. New York: Sage.

Saleh, L. D., & Operario, D. (2009). Beyond the "down low": A critical analysis of terminology guiding HIV prevention efforts with African American men who have sex with men. *Social Science & Medicine, 68*, 390–95.

Sandfort, T., & Dodge, B. (2008). And then there was the down low: Introduction to Black and Latino male bisexualities. *Archives of Sexual Behavior, 37*, 675–82.

Sanyal, P. (2009). From credit to collective action: The role of microfinance in promoting women's social capital and normative influence. *American Sociological Review, 74*, 529–50.

Sanyal, P. (2014). *Credit to Capabilities: A Sociological Study of Microcredit Groups in India*. London: Cambridge University Press.

Sareen, J., Pagura, J., & Grant, B. (2009). Is intimate partner violence associated with HIV infection among women in the United States? *General Hospital Psychiatry, 31*, 274–78.

Schuler, S. R., & Hashemi, S. M. (1994). Credit programs, women's empowerment, and contraceptive use in rural Bangladesh. *Studies in Family Planning, 25*, 65–76.

Schultz, A. J., & Mullings, L. (2006). *Gender, Race, & Class: Intersectional Approaches*. San Francisco: Jossey-Bass.

Scott, J. (1986). Gender: A useful category of historical analysis. *American Historical Review, 91*, 1053–75.

Seal, D., Wagner-Raphael, L. I., & Ehrhardt, A. A. (2000). Sex, intimacy, and HIV: An ethnographic study of a Puerto Rican social group in New York City. *Journal of Psychology & Human Sexuality, 11*, 51–92.

Seal, D. W., & Ehrhardt, A. A. (2003). Masculinity and urban men: Perceived scripts for courtship, romantic, and sexual interactions. *Culture, Health, & Sexuality, 5*, 295–319.

Seal, D. W., & Ehrhardt, A. A. (2004). HIV prevention–related sexual health promotion for heterosexual men in the United States: Pitfalls and recommendations. *Archives of Sexual Behavior, 33*, 211–22.

Seal, D. W., Exner, T. M., & Ehrhardt, A. A. (2003). HIV sexual risk reduction intervention with heterosexual men. *Archives of Internal Medicine, 153*, 738–39.

Segal, L. (1994). *Straight Sex: Rethinking the Politics of Pleasure*. Berkeley: University of California Press.

Seidman, G. (1999). Gendered citizenship: South Africa's democratic transition and the construction of a gendered state. *Gender & Society, 13*, 287–307.

Seidman, G. (2003). Institutional dilemmas: Representation versus mobilization in the South African Gender Commission. *Feminist Studies, 29*, 541–63.

Seidman, S. (2009). *The Social Construction of Sexuality*. New York: Norton.

Sen, G., & Grown, C. A. (1988). *Development, Crises, and Alternative Visions: Third World Women's Perspectives*. New York: Routledge.

Sengupta, R., & Aubuchon, C. P. (2008). The microfinance revolution: An overview. *Federal Reserve Bank of St. Louis Review, 90*, 9–30.

Serwadda, D., Gray, R., Wawer, M. J., Stallings, R. Y., Sewankambo, N. K., Konde-Lule, B., Lainjo, J. K., Kelly, R. (1995). The social dynamics of HIV transmission as reflected through discordant couples in rural Uganda. *AIDS, 9*, 745–50.

Shain, R. N., Piper, J. M., & Newton, E. R., et al. (1999). A randomized, controlled trial of a behavioral intervention to prevention sexually transmitted disease among minority women. *New England Journal of Medicine, 340*, 93–100.

Shefer, T., Crawford, M., Simbayi, L. C., Dwadha-Henda, N., Cloete, A., Kaufman, M., & Kalichman, S. (2008). Gender, power, and resistance to change among two communities in the Western Cape, South Africa. *Feminism and Psychology, 18*, 157–82.

Shefer, T., & Foster, D. (2009). Heterosex among young South Africans: Research reflections. Pp. 267–89 in in M. Steyn & M. van Zyl (eds.), *The Prize and the Price: Shaping Sexualities in South Africa*. Cape Town: HSRC Press.

Sherman, S. G., German, Y., Cheng, M., Marks, M., & Bailey-Kloche, M. (2006). The evaluation of the JEWEL project: An innovative economic-enhancement and HIV-prevention intervention study targeting drug-using women involved in prostitution. *AIDS Care, 18*, 1–11.

Shi, C. S., Kouyoumdjian, F. G., & Dushoff, J. (2013). Intimate partner violence is associated with HIV infection in Kenya. *BMC Public Health, 13*, doi: 10.1186/1471-2458-13-512.

Shisana, O., & Simbayi, L. (2008). *South African National HIV Prevalence, HIV Incidence, Behaviour, and Communication Survey, 2005*. Cape Town, South Africa: Human Sciences Research Council.

Sideris, T. (2004). You have to change and you don't know how! Contesting what it means to be a man in a rural area of South Africa. *Journal of African Studies, 63*, 29–49.

Siegel, K., Scrimshaw, E., Lekas, H. M., & Parsons, J. T. (2008). Sexual behaviors of non–gay-identified men who have sex with men and women. *Archives of Sexual Behavior, 37*, 720–35.

Sievers, M., & Vandenberg, P. (2007). Synergies through linkages: Who benefits from linking micro-finance and business development services? *World Development, 35*, 1341–58.

Sikkema, K., Kelly, J., Winett, R., Solomon, L., Cargill, V., Roffman, R., et al. (2000). Outcomes of a randomized community-level HIV-prevention intervention for women living in 18 low-income inner-city housing developments. *American Journal of Public Health, 90*, 57–63.

Silverman, J. G., et al. (2008). Intimate partner violence and HIV infection among married Indian women. *JAMA, 300*, 703–10.

Simoni, J. M., Walters, K. L., & Nero, D. K. (2000). Safer sex among HIV+ women: The role of relationships. *Sex Roles, 42*, 691–708.

Simpson, A. (2005). Sons and fathers/boys to men in the time of AIDS: Learning masculinity in Zambia. *Journal of Southern African Studies, 31*, 569–86.

Smoyer, A. B., & Patterson, H. R. (2007). *Can Microenterprise Programs Reduce HIV Risk in the United States? Policy Update*. New Haven: CT: Center for Interdisciplinary Research on AIDS.

Sobo, E. (1995). Finance, romance, social support, and condom use among impoverished inner-city women. *Human Organization, 54*, 115–28.

Somerville, S. B. (2000). *Queering the Color Line: Race and the Invention of Homosexuality in American Culture*. Durham, NC: Duke University Press.

Sonke Gender Justice Network (2007). One Man Can workshop activities: Talking to men about gender, sexual and domestic violence, and HIV/AIDS. Available at http://www.genderjustice.org.za/onemancan/completeone-man-can-toolkit/download-the-complete-to.html

Sonke Gender Justice Network (2012). You can't just fold your arms: Sonke Gender Justice's quest to transform men in post-apartheid South Africa. Available at http://vimeo.com/46332577

Spikes, P. S., Purcell, D. W., Williams, K. M., Chen, Y., Ding, H., & Sullivan, P. S. (2009). Sexual risk behaviors among HIV-positive Black men who have sex with women, with men, or with men and women: Implications for intervention development. *American Journal of Public Health, 99*, 1072–78.

Stacey, J., & Thorne, B. (1985). The missing feminist revolution in sociology. *Social Problems, 32*, 301–16.

Staples, R. (2006). *Exploring Black Sexuality*. Boulder, CO: Rowman & Littleton.

Statistics South Africa (2013). Key statistics: The economy. Available at beta2.statssa.gov.za.

Stein, Z. A. (1990). HIV prevention: The need for methods women can use. *American Journal of Public Health, 80*, 460–62.

Stern, O., Peacock, D., & Alexander, H. (2009). Working with men and boys: Emerging strategies from across Africa to address gender-based violence and HIV/AIDS. Sonke Gender Justice and the Men Engage Network. Available at www.sonkegenderjustice.org

Stewart, R., Rooyen, C., Dickson, K., Majoro, M., & Wet, T. (2010). What Is the Impact of Microfinance on Poor Oeople? A Systematic Review of Evidence from sub-Saharan Africa. London: EPPI-Centre, Social Science Research Unit, Institute of Education, University of London. Available at http://r4d.dfid.gov.uk/Output/185865/Default.aspx

Stokes, J. P., McKirnan, D. J., Doll, K., & Burzette, R. G. (1996). Female partners of bisexual men: What they don't know might hurt them. *Psychology of Women Quarterly, 20*, 267–84.

Stombler, M., Baunach, D. M., Burgess, E. O., Donnelly, D. J., Simonds, W. O., & Windsor, E. J. (eds.) (2009). *Sex Matters: The Sexuality and Society Reader*. Upper Saddle River, NJ: Pearson.

Stratford, D., Mizuno, Y., Williams, K., Courtenay-Quirk, C., & O'Leary, A. (2008). Addressing poverty as risk for disease: Recommendations from CDC's consultation on microenterprise as HIV prevention. *Public Health Reports, 123*, 9–20.

Strebel, A. (1995). Whose epidemic is it? Reviewing the literature on women and AIDS. *South African Journal of Psychology, 25*, 12–20.

Sumartojo, E., Doll, L., Holtgrave, D., Gayle, H., & Merson, M. (2000). Enriching the mix: Incorporating structural factors into HIV prevention. *AIDS, 14*, 1, S1–S2.

Swarr, A. (2012). *Sex in Transition: Remaking Gender & Race in South Africa*. New York: SUNY Press.

Tello, J., Cervantes, R. C., Cordova, D., & Santos, S. M. (2010). Joven Noble: Evaluation of a culturally focused youth development program. *Journal of Community Psychology, 38*, 799–811.

Teunis N. (2007). Sexual objectification and the construction of whiteness in the gay male community. *Culture, Health, and Sexuality, 9*, 263–75.

Thing, J. (2010). Gay, Mexican, and immigrant: Intersecting identities among gay men in Los Angeles. *Social Identities, 16*, 809–31.

Thomas, J. C., & Thomas, K. K. (1999). Things ain't what they ought to be: Social forces underlying racial disparities in rates of sexually transmitted diseases in a rural North Carolina county. *Social Science & Medicine, 49*, 1075–84.

Thompson, L. (2000). *A History of South Africa*. New Haven, CT: Yale University Press.

Thornton Dill, B. (1988). Our mother's grief: Racial ethnic women and the mainte- nance of families. *Journal of Family History, 13*, 415–31.

Thornton Dill, B., & Baca-Zinn, M. (1984). Difference and domination. Pp. 3–12 in B. Dill & M. Baca-Zinn (eds.), *Women of Color in U.S. Society*. Philadelphia: Temple University Press.

Tiefer, L. (1990). *Sex Is Not a Natural Act and Other Essays*. Boulder, CO: Westview.

Treichler, P. (1988). AIDS, gender, and biomedical discourse: Current contests for meaning. Pp. 190–266 in E. Fee & D. M. Fox (eds.), *AIDS: The Burden of History* Berkeley: University of California Press.

Treichler, P. (1999a). AIDS, homophobia, and biomedical discourse: An epidemic of signification. Pp. 190–266 in R. Parker & P. Aggleton (eds.), *Culture, Society, and Sexuality: A Reader*. Philadelphia: Taylor & Francis.

Treichler, P. (1999b). *How to Have Theory in an Epidemic: Cultural Chronicles of AIDS*. Durham, NC: Duke University Press.

Truth, S. (1851/2000). Ain't I a woman? Pp. 250–51 in E. Ashton-Jones, Gary A. Olson, & M. Perry (eds.), *The Gender Reader*. Boston: Allyn & Bacon.

Tsai, A., Hung, K. J., & Weiser, S. (2012). Is food insecurity associated with HIV risk? Cross-sectional evidence from sexually active women in Brazil. *PLoS Medicine*, DOI: 10.1371/journal.pmed.1001203.

Turner, W. (2000). *A Genealogy of Queer Theory*. Philadelphia: Temple University Press.

UNAIDS (2000). Men and AIDS: A gendered approach. 2000 World AIDS Campaign. Geneva, Switzerland. Available at http://data.unaids.org/pub/ report/2000/20000622_wac_men_en.pdf

UNAIDS (2001). Working with men for HIV prevention and care. Geneva, Switzer- land. Available at http://www.unaids.org

UNAIDS (2008). Report on the global epidemic. Available at http://www.unaids.org

UNAIDS (2011). Report on the global epidemic. Available at http://www.unaids.org

UNAIDS (2012). Report on the global epidemic. Available at http://www.unaids.org

United Nations Population Information Network (1994). Report on the international conference on population and development. Available at http://www.un.org/popin/ icpd/conference/offeng/poa.html

USDOJ (2006). Bureau of Justice Statistics bulletin: Prisoners. Available at http://www. ojp.usdoj.gov/bjs/pub/pdf/p06.pdf

Valocchi, S. (2007). Not yet queer enough: Lessons of queer theory for the sociology of gender and sexuality. *Gender & Society, 19*, 750–70.

Vance, C. S. (1983). Gender systems, ideology, and sex research. Pp. 371–84 in A. Snitow, C. Stansell, & S. Thompson (eds.), *Powers of Desire: The Politics of Sexuality*. New York: Monthly Review Press.

Vance, C. S. (1993). Pleasure and danger: Toward a politics of sexuality. Pp. 1–27 in C. S. Vance (ed.), *Pleasure and Danger: Exploring Female Sexuality*. Boston: Routledge.

Van den Berg, W., Godana, P., Hendricks, L., Hatcher, A., & Dworkin, S. L. (2013). Shifts in fatherhood beliefs and parenting practices following a gender-transformative health programme in Eastern Cape, South Africa. *Gender & Development, 21*, 111–25.

Van den Wingaard, M. (1997). *Reinventing the Sexes: The Biomedical Construction of Masculinity and Femininity*. Bloomington: Indiana University Press.

van Klinken, A. S. (2011). Male headship as male agency: An alternative understanding of a "patriarchal" African Pentecostal discourse on masculinity. *Religion & Gender, 1*, 104–24.

van Klinken, A. S. (2013a). Transforming masculinities towards gender justice in an era of HIV and AIDS: Plotting the pathways. Pp. 275–96 in *Transforming Masculinities towards Gender Justice in an Era of HIV and AIDS: Gender Controversies in Times of AIDS*. Surrey, UK: Ashgate.

van Klinken, A. S. (2013b). *Transforming Masculinities towards Gender Justice in an Era of HIV and AIDS: Gender Controversies in Times of AIDS*. Surrey, UK: Ashgate.

Venkata, N. A., & Yamini, V. (2010). Why do microfinance clients take multiple loans? MicroSave India Focus Note 33, February. Available at http://www.microsave.net/resource/why_do_microfinance_clients_take_multiple_loans#.VJmlUBoMNQ

Verma, R., Pulerwitz, J., Mahendra, V. S., Khandekar, S., Singh, S. K., Das, S. S., Mehra, S., & Nura, A. (2008). Promoting Gender Equity as a Strategy to Reduce HIV Risk and Gender-Based Violence among Young Men in India. Horizons Final Report. Washington, DC: Population Council. Available at http://www.popcouncil.org/pdfs/horizons/India_GenderNorms.pdf

Vittelone, N. (2000). Condoms and the making of "testosterone man": A cultural analysis of the male sex drive in AIDS research on safer heterosex. *Men & Masculinities, 3*, 152–67.

Voelker, R. (2008). Studies illuminate HIV's inequalities. *Journal of the American Medical Association, 299*, 269–75.

Wagner, L. I., Seal, D. W., & Ehrhardt, A. A. (2001). Close emotional relationships with women versus men: A qualitative study of 56 heterosexual men living in an inner-city neighborhood. *Journal of Men's Studies, 9*, 243–56.

Waldby, C. (1996). *AIDS and the Body Politic: Biomedicine and Sexual Difference*. London: Routledge.

Waldron, I. (1995). Contributions of changing gender differences in behavior and social roles to changing gender differences in mortality. Pp. 22–45 in D. Sabo & D. F. Gordon (eds.), *Men's Health and Illness: Gender, Power, and the Body*. New York: Sage.

Walker, L. (2005). Men behaving differently: South African men since 1994. *Culture, Health, Sexuality, 7*, 225–38.

Walker, L., Reid, G., & Cornell, M. (eds.) (2004). *Waiting to Happen: HIV/AIDS in South Africa [The Bigger Picture]*. London: Reiner.

Warner, M. (1993). *Fear of a Queer Planet*. Minneapolis: University of Minnesota Press.

Watts, C. H., & May, R. (1992). The influence of concurrent partnerships on the dynamics of HIV/AIDS. *Mathematical Bioscience, 108*, 89–104.

Watts, C. H., & Zimmerman, C. (2002). Violence against women: Global scope and magnitude, *Lancet, 359*, 1232–37.

Watkins-Hayes, C. (2014). Intersectionality and the sociology of HIV/AIDS: Past, present, and future research directions. *Annual Review of Sociology, 40*, 431–57.

Weeks, J. (1985). *Sexuality and Its Discontents: Meanings, Myths, and Modern Sexualities*. New York: Routledge.

Weeks, J. (2002). *Sexuality*. London: Routledge.

Wegner, M. N., Landry, E., Wilkinson, D., & Tzanis, J. Men as partners in reproductive health. *International Family Planning Perspectives, 24*. Available at https://www.guttmacher.org/pubs/journals/2403898.html

Weinberg, M. S., Williams, C. J., & Pryor, D. W. (1994). *Dual Attraction: Understanding Bisexuality*. New York: Oxford University Press.

Weiser, S., et al. (2007). Food insufficiency is associated with high-risk sexual behavior among women in Botswana and Swaziland. *PLoS Medicine, 4*, 1589–97.

Weiser, S. D., Leiter, K., Bangsberg, D. R., Kegeles, S., Ragland, K. R., Kushel, M. B., & Frongillo, E. A. (2009). Food insecurity among homeless and marginally housed individuals living with HIV/AIDS in San Francisco. *AIDS & Behavior, 13*, 841–48.

Weiss, E., & Gupta, G. R. (1998). *Bridging the Gap: Addressing Gender and Sexuality in HIV Prevention*. Washington, DC: International Center for Research on Women.

West, C., & Fenstermaker, S. (1995). Doing difference. *Gender & Society, 9*, 8–37.

West, C., & Zimmerman, D. H. (1987). Doing gender. *Gender and Society, 1*, 125–51.

Wheeler, D. P., et al. (2008). A comparative analysis of sexual risk characteristics of black men who have sex with men or women and men. *Archives of Sexual Behavior, 37*, 697–707.

White V., Greene, M., & Murphy, E. (2003). Men and Reproductive Health Programs: Influencing Gender Norms. Washington, DC: Synergy Project. Available at http://www.synergyaids.com/SynergyPublications/Gender_Norms.pdf

WHO (2000). Violence against women and HIV/AIDS: Setting the research agenda. Geneva. Available at http://www.who.int/gender/violence/VAWhiv.pdf

WHO (2004). Violence against women and HIV/AIDS: Critical Intersections. Geneva. Available at http://whqlibdoc.who.int/unaids/2004/a85591.pdf?ua=1

WHO (2005). Garcia-Moreno, C., Jansen, H. A. F. M., Ellsberg, M., Heise, L., Watts, C. H. WHO multi-country study on women's health and domestic violence against women: Initial results on prevalence, health outcomes, and women's responses. Available online.

WHO (2013). Violence against women: Intimate partner and sexual violence against women. Available at http://www.who.int/mediacentre/factsheets/fs239/en

Williams, C. A. (1999). *Roman Homosexuality*. Oxford: Oxford University Press.

Williams, S. P., Gardos, P. S., Ortiz-Torres, B., Tross, S., & Ehrhardt, A. A. (2001). Urban women's negotiation strategies for safer sex with their male partners. *Women & Health, 33*, 133–48.

Wilson, W. J. (1987). *The Truly Disadvantaged: The Inner City, the Underclass, and Public Policy*. Chicago: University of Chicago Press.

Wilson, W. J. (1996). *When Work Disappears: The World of the New Urban Poor*. New York: Vintage.

Wilton, T. (1994). Silences, absences, and fragmentation. Pp. 1–6 in L. Doyal, J. Naidoo, & T. Wilton (eds.), *AIDS: Setting a Feminist Agenda*. London: Taylor & Francis.

Wilton, T., & Aggleton, P. (1990). Young People and Safer Sex. Paper presented at the First Scandinavian Conference on Safer Sex, Stockholm, Sweden.

Wingood, G. M., & DiClemente, R. J. (1996). HIV sexual risk reduction interventions for women: A review. *American Journal of Preventative Medicine, 12*, 209–17.

Wingood, G. M., & DiClemente, R. J. (2000). Application of the theory of gender and power to examine HIV-related exposures, risk factors, and effective interventions for women. *Health Education & Behavior, 27*, 539–65.

Wingood, G. M., & DiClemente, R. J. (2002). The theory of gender and power: A social structural theory for guiding public health interventions. Pp. 313–46 in R. J. DiClemente, R. A. Crosby, & M. C. Kegler (eds.), *Emerging Theories in Health Promotion Practice and Research*. San Francisco: Jossey-Bass.

Wingood, G. M., DiClemente, R. J., Mikhail, I., et al. (2004). A randomized controlled trial to reduce HIV/AIDS transmission among women living with HIV: The Willow Program. *Journal of Acquired Immune Deficiency Syndromes, 37*, S58–S67.

Wingood, G. M., DiClemente, R. J., Villamizar, K., Er, D., DeVarona, M., Taveras, J., Jean, R. (2011). Efficacy of a health-educator-delivered HIV-prevention intervention for Latina women: A randomized controlled trial. *American Journal of Public Health, 101*, 2245–52.

Wingood, G. M., Simpson-Robinson, L., Braxton, N., & Raiford, J. L. (2013). Design of a faith-based HIV intervention: Successful collaboration between a university and a church. *Health Promotion Practice, 12*, 823–31.

Wingood, G. M., et al. (2013). Comparative effectiveness of a faith-based HIV intervention for African-American women: Importance of enhancing religious social capital. *American Journal of Public Health, 103*, 2226–33. Available online.

Wolitski, R., the Project Start Writing Group, & the Project Start Study Group (2006). Relative efficacy of a multi-session sexual-risk reduction for young men released from prisons in 4 states. *American Journal of Public Health, 96*, 1854–61.

Wood, K., & Jewkes, R. (1997). Violence, rape, and sexual coercion: Everyday love in a South African township. *Gender and Development, 5*, 41–46.

Wright, T. C. Jr., Ellerbrock, T. V., Chiasson, M. A., Van Devanter, N., & Sun, X. W. (1994). Cervical intraepithelial neoplasia in women infected with Human Immunodeficiency Virus: Prevalence, risk factors, and validity of Papanicolaou smears. New York Cervical Disease Study. *Obstetrics & Gynecology, 84*, 591–97.

Wyrod, R. (2008). Beyond women's rights and men's authority: Masculinity and shifting discourses of gender difference in urban Uganda. *Gender & Society, 22*, 799–823.

Wyrod, R. (2016). *Privilege in a Plague: AIDS and the Remaking of Masculinity*. Berkeley: University of California Press.

Young, R. M., & Meyer, I. (2005). The trouble with "MSM" and "WSW": Erasure of the sexual-minority person in public health discourse. *American Journal of Public Health, 95*, 1144–49.

Yunus, M. (2003). *Banker to the Poor: Micro-Lending and the Battle against World Poverty*. New York: Public Affairs Press.

Zierler, S. (1997). Hitting hard: HIV and violence. Pp. 207–21 in N. Goldstein & J. L. Manlowe (eds.), *The Gender Politics of HIV/AIDS in Women*. New York: New York University Press.

Zierler, S., & Krieger, N. (1997). Reframing women's risk: Social inequalities and HIV infection. *Annual Review of Public Health, 18*, 401–36.

Zukoski, A., & Cupples, J. B. (2008). *Male Advocates for Responsible Sexuality (MARS) Program Final Report (2003-2008)*. Corvallis, OR: Benton County Health Department.

INDEX

ABOUT THE AUTHOR

Shari L. Dworkin is Professor of Sociology in the Department of Social and Behavioral Sciences and Associate Dean for Academic Affairs at the University of California–San Francisco School of Nursing. She is the author of over sixty journal articles focused on gender, sexuality, and health. She is author or editor of several books, most recently *Women's Empowerment and Global Health: A 21st-Century Agenda* (forthcoming), coedited with Monica Gandhi and Paige Passano, and *Body Panic: Gender, Health, and the Selling of Fitness* (2009), also with New York University Press.